general practice
the uncertain art

general practice
the uncertain art

JOHN STEVENS

MCGRAW-HILL BOOK COMPANY Sydney
New York San Francisco Auckland Bogotá
Caracas Lisbon London Madrid Mexico City
Milan Montreal New Delhi San Juan
Singapore Tokyo Toronto

McGraw·Hill Australia
A Division of The **McGraw·Hill** *Companies*

Text © 1999 Dr John Stevens
Illustrations and design © 1999 McGraw-Hill Book Company Australia Pty Limited
Additional owners of copyright are named in on-page credits.

Apart from any fair dealing for the purposes of study, research, criticism or review, as permitted under the *Copyright Act*, no part may be reproduced by any process without written permission. Enquiries should be made to the publisher, marked for the attention of the Permissions Editor, at the address below.

Every effort has been made to trace and acknowledge copyright material. Should any infringement have occurred accidentally the authors and publishers tender their apologies.

Copying for educational purposes
Under the copying provisions of the *Copyright Act*, copies of parts of this book may be made by an educational institution. An agreement exists between the Copyright Agency Limited (CAL) and the relevant educational authority (Department of Education, university, TAFE, etc.) to pay a licence fee for such copying. It is not necessary to keep records of copying except where the relevant educational authority has undertaken to do so by arrangement with the Copyright Agency Limited.

For further information on the CAL licence agreements with educational institutions, contact the Copyright Agency Limited, Level 19, 157 Liverpool Street, Sydney NSW 2000. Where no such agreement exists, the copyright owner is entitled to claim payment in respect of any copies made.

Enquiries concerning copyright in McGraw-Hill publications should be directed to the Permissions Editor at the address below.

National Library of Australia Cataloguing-in-Publication data:

Stevens, John, (John Alfred)
General practice: the uncertain art.

ISBN 0 07 470725 6.

1. Stevens, John, John Alfred. 2. Physicians (General practice) – Australia – Biography. 3. Physicians (General practice) – Australia. 4. Rural health – Australia. I. Title

610.92

Published in Australia by
McGraw-Hill Book Company Australia Pty Limited
4 Barcoo Street, Roseville NSW 2069, Australia
Acquisitions Editor: Kristen Baragwanath
Production Editors: Sybil Kesteven, Caroline Hunter
Designer: Jenny Pace Design
Cover design: Jenny Pace Design
Cover illustrator: Alison Wallace, Lonely Badger
Typeset in 9pt Belwe by Jenny Pace Design
Printed on 80 gsm Woodfree by
Best-Tri Colour Printing & Packaging, Co. Ltd, Hong Kong

'You arrive palpitating [at the emergency scene] . . . and the crowd parts respectfully to watch the professional hero in action. You clutch your bag in self-defence—it's usually about the right height and weight for discouraging Alsatians, although Corgis can slip underneath and nip you—and wonder what the hell to do.'

'I drew up to the house . . . and reached into the boot with practised ease for my bag. It wasn't there. I felt extraordinarily naked walking up the garden path with no bag to swing, no badge of office, no staff of therapeutic comfort or wand of diagnostic magic. She had sent for me and, poor girl, that's all she got.'

'We are not gatekeepers. How can we be when there are so many gaps in the fence on either side?'

Quotations such as these from this delightful book present the unique literary flair of John Stevens, a legendary figure for two decades to the readers of *Australian Family Physician* (*AFP*), the journal of the Royal Australian College of General Practitioners. John attracted a following of adoring colleagues as the witty, erudite author of 'On the level' and 'Item 1'—regular up front features in *AFP*.

It was my privilege as medical editor of *AFP* to work closely with this very genial and humble man and encourage him to muster his weary resources at the end of the day to maintain his monthly column. As he would say, 'the sands of weekend freedom trickle remorselessly by'. When he eventually hung up his pen in 1994, his legion of fans were very disappointed. His thought-provoking articles had stimulated, stirred and amused.

I am therefore pleased to be writing a foreword to a collection of his writings under a most appropriate and characteristic Stevenian title, *General Practice: The Uncertain Art*.

A profile in the *AFP* series 'Notable Australian Doctors' reads, 'Dr John Stevens approaches his work as a GP in Tasmania with passion and integrity. The dual love of literature and medicine has provided the basis of a philosophy of life for this energetic and talented man'.

John attributes his love of literature to his father reading him tales of Dickens when he was a small boy. His father was a facilitator who 'kindled a spark that is burning still'. Born in London, John was educated at Epsom College and then London University, gaining his medical degree in 1954. His postgraduate work included service as a flight lieutenant in the Royal Air Force medical branch and posts in a number of hospitals. He gained his D Obst RCOG in 1959 and after six years in general practice in Biggin Hill, Kent, moved to Tasmania where he has been, in Ulverstone, for over thirty years.

His writings in this book reveal a deeply human understanding of his patients and his calling:

'. . . the language of our patients is a thing of vernacular and euphemism, allusion and obsolete belief. How many lay words can you list for defecation or menstruation? What bizarre symptomatology (pointless, pompous word that it is) cannot a virus cause? What anxiety lies behind a reference to the "old ticker"?'

His long experience as a family doctor has led to wise and humble reflections.

'Time and disaster have humbled the brash young medical officer of more than thirty years ago. I have learnt to qualify my certainties, temper my enthusiasms and mute my prophecies. I know, if nothing else, that nothing is quite so bad or so good as it seems at first and that the cost of my mistakes is borne by others, though the memories of them are mine alone.'

The liberal use of quotations from John Stevens' *General Practice: The Uncertain Art* in this foreword conveys the richness and humour awaiting those who are fortunate enough to possess this book. I applaud McGraw-Hill Book Company Australia for having the foresight to publish it.

John Murtagh
Professor of General Practice
Department of Community Medicine and General Practice
Monash University

the author

JOHN STEVENS was born in England in 1931. He was educated at Epsom College and graduated from Guys Hospital, London, in 1954. After completing the obligatory residencies, he entered the RAF and served for three years as a Medical Officer prior to undertaking further hospital posts as a prelude to entering general practice in the UK in 1959. In 1964, after some six years in partnership practice, he migrated with his wife Mary and their three children to join a fellow Guys man in Ulverstone, Tasmania, in the practice from which he eventually retired in 1994.

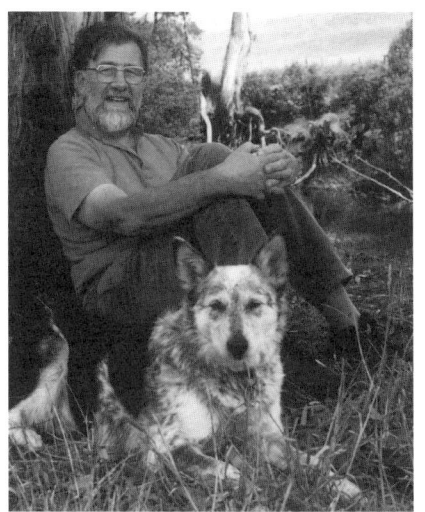

He was first drawn into the RACGP in 1966 and has been involved with it in some capacity since. His involvement has included posts as a Council Member, State Provost, State Censor, member of the Examination Board and interest in undergraduate teaching.

Stevens' major contribution has been in the field of medical publications. He not only sat on the Board that originally set up the *Australian Family Physician*, but he also contributed an article to the inaugural edition. Thereafter he provided a monthly column, appearing under various titles, which ceased in 1993. He also edited a number of College publications including the handbook and *The Organisation of Family Practice*. In 1997, he delivered the annual William Connolly oration at the RACGP National Conference in Hobart.

Now retired, he divides his time between carpentry, fishing, golf and fiddling with the computer. He retains links with the profession as a member of both the Cancer Council of Tasmania and the state RACGP examination panel and by performing occasional odd jobs for the local Division of General Practice.

dedication

To the patients and partners who taught me my trade and to that special partner in life without whose constant help and endless patience I could never have practised it.

The general practitioner's professional reading is divided, like Gaul, into three parts: what they have to read; what they ought to read and what they'd rather read. It was with this latter category in mind that I first contributed an article to the initial number of *Australian Family Physician* in 1971. And thanks to the journal's unfailing encouragement and support, I have invaded their columns and imperilled their schedules on and off for some twenty-seven years.

It is a pleasure to record my appreciation of the tolerance of so many editors and the patience of so many editorial assistants with my irreverence and blithe disregard of deadlines and to acknowledge, with gratitude, the Editorial Board's permission to reisssue some of the articles which originally appeared in that journal as 'College Column', 'Item One' and latterly 'On the Level'.

I have been fortunate too in being able to persuade McGraw-Hill in the person of John Rowe in accepting (after some pardonable hesitation) the onus of publication and to their editorial and production staff, in particular Kristen Baragwanath in Melbourne and Sybil Kesteven in Sydney for their professional expertise and personal encouragement.

Many of the original articles were, of course, ephemeral, concerned with issues now resolved and problems no longer relevant but some I dare to think glance at more enduring matters: it is a selection of these that are here presented.

That they may be prejudiced, ill-considered or irrational is simply to show that they are one man's picture of this, the human face of medical practice. But however smart the technology, however well researched the process when I, the doctor, face you, the patient, it is only ourselves that really matter—my knowledge such as it is, your unease and our uncertainties in this the changeless, changing, shifting, enduring enterprise of *General Practice: The Uncertain Art*.

contents

v foreword
vii the author

introduction
3 the uncertain art
5 everybody's bastard
7 the doctor's glossary

getting there
13 on the selection of medical students
15 as she is spoke
18 my dear osbert
22 euhemeroi

being there
29 doctor in the wrong house
31 it's all in the bag
34 gladys
36 sick friends
38 gotcha
41 monday, bloody monday
43 the doctor tells
47 my colleague from the congo
49 the copper bracelet
51 giving it away
54 one eye on the cook
57 in at the death

give me my staff
63 give me my staff
66 none other than
68 but i don't want a nice day
71 letters pray

off and away

- 77 time off
- 79 'you was away'
- 82 why fishing?
- 85 anti-social climbing
- 87 overseas and overspent
- 89 small change
- 93 more than a month of sundays

but am i right?

- 99 because it's there
- 101 a question of responsibility
- 104 signs for all times
- 107 who says?
- 110 advice and consent
- 113 good grief
- 115 here at the gate
- 118 the middle ground
- 121 the impotent doctor
- 123 shocks and starts
- 126 talking shop
- 129 supermarket medicine
- 130 a view from the sticks
- 134 quality street
- 137 on second thoughts
- 140 a plague on all our houses

valedictory

- 145 valedictory

———————— introduction

the uncertain art ─────────────────────────

everybody's bastard ───────────────────────

─ the doctor's glossary ─────────────────────

the uncertain art

If you are the kind of person who likes labelling—most of us find it easier than thinking—you have somewhere in your mind a cerebral ticket office. Here, as each parcel is presented, you slap on the appropriate sticker, toss it onto the appropriate shelf and store unopened until the next parcel arrives.

Occasionally, accident or curiosity discloses quite unexpected contents and you are forced to re-label and place the parcel with the 'even thoughs': 'Even though he's in the tax office, he plays off three'; 'even though they live in Canberra ...' and so on (I've yet to hear it applied to a politician). It's a slightly disturbing process, being obliged to reconsider your judgments, but happily the 'even though' principle leaves your basic prejudices ingrained, like dirt.

Most professions have their epithets, which are usually included in a phrase that begins 'of course, he's a ...', or 'what else would you expect from a ...'. We slash happily at our tall poppies and lean enviously on the fences of greener pastures, bigger incomes and easier lives. Lawyers have 'keen legal minds' if they're on our side, or are 'pettifoggers' (lovely word) if they're not. Accountants are 'accurate' if the tax demand is low, 'unenterprising' if it is not. Politicians lie, teachers laze and parsons drone.

But what do GPs do? Sign things—anything say the lawyers. Forget things—everything say the newspapers. Overlook things—vital things say other doctors.

My kinder word is compromise. The whole process of caring involves adaptation: adapting the patient to the pathology; modifying the treatment to the treated; replacing the broadsides of fashionable prevention with a single shot at a moving and elusive bulls eye.

You have to preach an often-changing gospel to a seldom-changing sceptic, who alters habits with reluctance, if at all. And, you have to accept the consequences of your failures.

You may well convince a smoker that a single puff spells doom, but can you then assure him that this cough, that bizarre sensation in the lower ribs, is not necessarily the first blast of the last trumpet? Can you impress on the unalterable obese that a minor rise in lipid minimoles does not presage imminent collapse at the breakfast table, or that lumbar backache is unlikely to be anginal? In short, are you good enough to handle the phobias created by your own preventive zeal?

Cardiac surgeons might logically abandon those who spoil their handiwork by refusing to reform. Orthopods could direct AIDS sufferers to other more expendable agencies. I have absolutely no evidence to suggest that either happens, but at the last we cannot choose our patients. We must compromise.

A homily delivered once may strike home, repeated twice may bear eventual fruit, but endlessly reiterated it simply drives the victim angrily away.

Herein lies our greatest danger: in modifying the message, it may at last be given no more. In descending from the pulpit we may join the congregation slumbering below. In tailoring a diuretic regimen to a social program, the patient may be grateful, but the myocardium is not. For abandoning the pursuit of normotension there may be a price to pay in speechless immobility and a vegetable life of bed pans and bed sores. A price not paid by us, the GPs.

C. S. Lewis once described a minister as spending so long in watering down the faith for his parishioners that it was he who shocked them by his unbelief. Do I see myself?

So we spend our working lives on a therapeutic tightrope, the level of which is now and then abruptly altered by the experts. We learn the hard way that trust, not affection, is the core, and understanding and mutual respect the essence. We learn to talk of chances, not statistics. A two-to-one chance of recovery sounds much more hopeful than a mortality rate of 33.3 per cent. We have to temper our therapeutic enthusiasms with reality and transmit our preventive messages with discretion.

We recognise that conclusions reached at the New England Baptist may not apply at the local hospital and that most advances trumpeted in the tabloids, or detailed in depth by the digests, sometimes prove more illusory than real. Indeed, next week or next month, a no less spectacular reverse may be gleefully disseminated by the same organs.

If we ever have a GP anthem I would propose an old wartime chorus:

> Treat 'em all,
> Treat 'em all,
> The fat and the slack and the tall,
> The overweight smokers who drive everywhere,
> The vitamised joggers who don't wash their hair,
> And those with no notion,
> Of fitness promotion,
> Come cheer up my lads treat 'em all.

We can you know, if we compromise.

everybody's bastard

There is something melancholy about Sundays. The sands of weekend freedom trickle remorselessly away and another working week comes round, predictably unpredictable, certainly uncertain. You shed the casual garments of release, reload your working pockets with pens and keys and credit cards and steal a glance at next week's diary. You put away the tools and toys and wonder where the endless leisure that beckoned on Friday night has gone. If the following weekend is a duty one the plodding journey to your next escape is bleak indeed.

It is a time for serious reflection and, should you have an article to write, an invitation to morbidity. Your natural resilience is heavily involved with the digestive overload of Sunday lunch, leaving only a dull autumnal prospect of decay.

It is then that my thoughts turn to epitaphs and obituaries and I wonder what they'll say about me later on.

It's not all that difficult to predict. I've sat through enough funeral sermons, all apparently about the same person, to sketch out my own. There will be a list of doings and achievements, whose accuracy depends solely on the recollections or briefing of the orator, an emphasis on virtues that visibly astonish the audience and a word of comfort to the survivors. There is a stern inquiry of death—where is its victory, where grave its sting (or is it the other way around?), a wobbly 23rd Psalm, if you're unlucky *Amazing Grace*, and then the mourners file out into the sunshine, discreetly confident of their own immortality.

Later on, you may rate an obituary. Colleagues will learn, with some surprise, that 'beneath that somewhat forbidding manner, those who knew you discerned a generous heart'. Which they will rightly interpret as, although in general sullen and contemptuous, you had been detected occasionally in acts of common courtesy.

Or it may be that you were 'never too busy not to listen to your patients', which somehow implies that you were too busy to do anything else for them, and that your loved ones, eventually tiring of cold casseroles and overcooked vegetables, left your dinner in the oven and went their separate ways. You may find your involvement with this college or that society detailed and applauded and conjure up a picture of the committed committee goer endlessly prolonging dull meetings with duller speeches and, what is worse, rehearsing them at home.

But how would you like to be remembered? What pithy epitaph would you choose to enliven a Sunday stroll through the cemetery? What, after all, can you point to from Valhalla?

Most of your achievements, if achievements there are, are negative. The bone mended (God saw to that), the catastrophe averted or postponed, but how can you know and who but your colleagues understand your part in it.

It was written of Sir Christopher Wren, 'If you seek a monument look around you'—but that was in St Pauls. Written on a GP's tombstone, it would scarcely pass in a cemetery—however grimly accurate it might be.

I read somewhere of a doctor who directed that a bell should hang over his grave, so that if anyone rang he wouldn't get up. Mindful of that heartsinking phrase, 'While you're here doctor', I have long cherished a simple line above me, 'Not here any more'.

But I've a better one than that now.

It was suggested to me by a patient confined to bed by a hot lumbar disc. That is, a man physically fit but incapacitated, robbed of sleep, burdened by pain, frustrated by obligatory immobility and irritated by the limitations of treatment.

I called on him regularly for a while and, as it happened, usually at the same hour of the day. It didn't take long for me to become part of the monotonous routine of his confinement and when one day I was delayed, there came a telephone call: was I coming, and when?

I went, sat beside his bed and tried to delude us both that his straight leg raising was a little higher, his pain level a little lower. Then I explained my delay. That morning for me had involved a casualty at the hospital, a ventricular fibrillation at home and various other manifestations of Murphy's Law.

He accepted this in silence and then broke into the first smile of our association.

'Yes', he said, 'You're everybody's bastard, aren't you?'

That'll do for me—especially on Sunday nights.

the doctor's glossary

For those who, like me, try to keep up.

accreditation *n.* inspection of premises and records by unfamiliar colleagues (*see also* peer review).

authority *n.* high level (clerk) permission to prescribe departmentally unfavoured drugs.

benefit *n.* monies paid by government (a) *social*, to patients or (b) *medical*, to doctors, and returned by both as income tax.

cholesterol *n.* injurious metabolites, of value only to private pathologists and arid manufacturers of table margarine.

columnist *n.* disreputable hack employed and occasionally paid to separate journal articles from reviews and correspondence (*see also* gadfly, plagiarist, etc).

community *n.* originally discovered by psychiatrists wishing to discharge patients, this unmapped territory is being increasingly developed by the profession. Early explorers, notably those general practitioners who still did house calls, paved the way for systematic exploitation of the resources and usually friendly natives. Now visited regularly by nursing patrols and sporadic expeditions of specialists in search of clinical material and the legendary 'public image', which is said to be situated there.

The adjectival form of the word is used in the sense of 'pertaining to others', viz. (a) *community resources*, other people's money, (b) *community involvement*, other people's time, and (c) *community spirit*, other people's good nature.

conference *n.* annual meeting of doctors (a) *national*, Australian doctors in Fiji, (b) *international*, Fijian doctors in Melbourne and (c) *world*, American doctors anywhere.

dilatation *n.* a common subject of debate between obstetricians and midwives.

The verb is 'dilate' not 'dilatate', e.g. 'She's almost fully dilated doctor' or (simultaneously) 'She's nowhere near ready sister'.

The current trends to Caesarean section and home delivery, and sometimes both in the same case, may well render the term obsolete.

discipline *n.* heterogeneous and disorganised coterie of those united only by the same training and their suspicion of other disciplines.

drug (a) *traveller n.* unwelcome purveyor of needless samples and useless literature (b) *representative n.* honoured and welcome bearer of invitations to free entertainment and hand cream for ancillary staff.

empathy *n.* vicarious experience of another person's symptoms, e.g. 'I'm sick of people vomiting'; also, sympathetic exchange of symptoms and remedies between patient and doctor.

examination *n.* method of exclusion of manifestly unfit colleagues or obviously fit patients.

group *n.* a noun of association (a) *group discussion*, eight tongue-tied strangers in diffident pursuit of the obvious, (b) *group therapy*, a number of unhappy patients talking to each other while their therapist talks to him/herself, (c) *group learning situations*, what older physicians knew as a 'teaching round' and Hippocrates as 'shifting dullness'.

interaction *n.* two people talking about the same thing at the same time. Should one become silent at any stage, the other is said to be *holding dialogue* with him (the situation has no feminine equivalent). On the rare occasions when both listen, it is said to be *'meaningful'*. Interactions involving more than two are said to be *'at all levels'*, and those lasting longer than one hour are *'in-depth'*.

interface *n.* the place where interactions occur, e.g. the door of the consulting room, the hospital car park or the locker room of the golf club.

interflora *n.* seems to have slipped in by mistake.

motivation *n.* that inner conviction that induces others to do what you want. The reflexive form 'self-motivation' is a transient state, usually precipitated by guilt, fear or tax deductibility.

paramedical *n.* trained ancillary staff to whom tedious or insoluble problems are thankfully referred (*see also* therapist).

peer review *n.* inspection of premises and records by only too familiar colleagues (*see also* accreditation).

relaxation *n.* the art of avoiding continuing education. Embraces golf, sailing, horticulture or any other pleasurable activity except attendance at football matches, which is more correctly termed 'sports medicine'.

report *n.* explosive noise caused by requests for information from employers, lawyers or insurance companies.

session *n.* unit of time employed by statutory health authorities, roughly equivalent to the distance between one's private rooms and the private hospital.

Note that in academic circles 'time' is the more appropriate term, e.g. *'part time'* refers to those who are on study leave for six months of the year and *'full time'* to those who are away on sabbatical leave the entire year.

Note also *plenary session*, the conclusion of a seminar (see below), at which the front rows pass votes of thanks and the back rows exchange addresses and promise to keep in touch.

seminar *n.* series of lectures interrupted by hospitality paid for by all but the lecturers.

symposium *n.* lavish hospitality interrupted by occasional lectures paid for by pharmaceutical companies.

therapist *n.* one who treats people, without recourse to medicine or surgery. Common examples are (a) *physio*, by machinery, (b) *occupational*, by basketwork, (c) *psycho*, by talk, (d) *speech*, by signs, (e) *remedial*, by carpet bowls and (f) *diversional*, by bingo.

When a group of therapists meets to disagree about any given problem, they are said to be employing the 'team approach'. When they unite in criticism of the doctor they are termed 'allied health professionals'.

veteran *n.* an underprivileged survivor of battle who is denied the right to pay for medical care, prevailing mortgage rates or, in the last extremity, tax on motor cars (*see also* repat and TPI).

worker *n.* (a) *social*, a poorly paid individual who helps the homeless, luckless, feckless and witless with the aid of a telephone and a university degree, (b) *welfare*, as previous, but without the university degree.

——————————— getting there

on the selection of medical students ─────────────

as she is spoke ─────────────────────────

my dear osbert ──────────────────────────

euhemeroi ───────────────────────────────

on the selection of medical students

It's a year or two since I attended my selection interview to enter medicine. I had stumbled through an uncomprehended physics syllabus—I have never found my ignorance of Fleming's Right Hand Rule to be a serious professional disadvantage; was on nodding terms with the lilies of the field (*Lilliaceae*); could recite the mouth parts of the cockroach; and could draw the structural formula of phenol. More to the point, I was a sound, if unspectacular, front row forward and had recently contributed a solo part to what must have been the worst performance of Bach's Fifth Brandenburg Concerto that even a school orchestra could perpetrate.

The Dean presided. He was a formidable ex-rugby international with a black patch over one eye, which periodically dropped to reveal a weeping empty socket. It had a discouraging effect on nervous candidates. On his left, a court physician watched with languid disdain and on his right, the secretary of the Medical School unobtrusively masterminded the whole operation. They asked me, 'Why medicine?' I replied that I didn't know. (Previously rehearsed speeches about 'suffering humanity' wouldn't, I felt, go down well here.) Was I making a terrible mistake? I hoped not. So did they, no doubt. The Dean discussed rugby and the physician, to whom I had hesitatingly mentioned the Bach, drifted into a monologue on Baroque music. That, I suspect, clinched it. Anyway, later I received a letter of acceptance, along with a list of books and the address of an articulator of skeletons. I was launched.

The point of this tedious reminiscence is not that this form of selection is desirable (after all, it produced me), but when I later mixed with colleagues who had been selected by elaborate intelligence testing—by academic pre-eminence, by sporting prowess or sheer nepotism—they were not noticeably different.

In short, I suspect that it does not matter a damn how medical students are selected. Given the intelligence or application to clear whatever scholastic hurdles are fashionable, whether it be Latin prose, differential calculus or callisthenics, the absence of overt psychosis or a criminal record and the presence of considerable determination, why not pick them at random?

Exploration of motives is on the whole, I think, unwise. A number of those who set out to help others end up by helping themselves: dedicated would-be surgeons end up in public health, heavy drinkers turn into ascetic neurologists, the notably level-headed embrace psychiatry. Chance and poverty mould more careers than we like to admit. It seems that we cream off the top of the matriculation pot and restrict entry to the mathematically gifted. Is this, I wonder, why so many otherwise brilliant students seem semi-literate? They have all the gifts but expression. Should we really surrender the right of selecting our future colleagues to examiners in matriculation mathematics?

Medicine is fashionable and relatively lucrative. It demands application and intelligence. It draws on all of one's resources except, perhaps, the creative. But it does not require that every doctor should be superman/woman. Nor does it require that every applicant should be a genius and/or a saint.

Entry to medical courses has become the ultimate school prize, the accolade awarded to the winners of a long and exhausting academic battle. We may be getting the best, but the best what? We should find room for the lazy, whose interests once caught, drive them to the top. There should be a place for those who study what the older universities accurately call the humanities. We could all do with a few poets and peasants.

If schoolmasters are not to pick our future colleagues, still less should the psychologists. It is difficult enough for doctors to agree on their own essential attributes. How can they explain to anyone else what they're looking for? Let's leave the inkblots out of this. My suggestion is an agreed educational standard that would exclude the dullards, an above average desire to enter medicine and a selection committee composed of the learned, the wise and the sensible in our profession. We must ensure that they do not choose too many replicas of the Dean (a hideous eventuality) and only those nephews and nieces that are truly deserving, and then leave them to it.

It would be a post of honour and some danger, but we would at least retain some control over our own future.

And if that system fails, why not pick the names out of the Dean's hat?

It should be big enough.

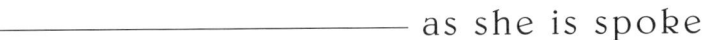

as she is spoke

'These results considered with some other recent reports suggest that academic success in a medical course is predicted to a surprisingly high level by competence in English. Both the importance of communication skills to the practice of medicine, and their assessment in those seeking entry to medical schools, are considered.'[1]

Why 'surprisingly'? That the best able to understand (and listen to) their patients and the most skilful in conveying their consequent opinion are more likely to perceive the problem, explain the cause and outline the solution, would, I should have thought, been obvious, even to an academic. There is a special pleasure in seeing another mount our cherished hobbyhorse; a peculiar thrill when a voice crying in the wilderness raises a distant echo.

For the clinician, science is a tool, but language is a workshop. We must have to hand a physical chisel, a chemical plan, a biological guide. There is a continuing need for mathematical constants against which to measure the inconstant variables of sick humanity, some sort of logical premises (excuse the pun) in or on which to work, but interpretation and communication demand other skills. Why select doctors on criteria designed for engineers and physicists?

The medieval university, which I was just too young to attend, exercised its students in only three subjects, three indispensable attributes for the pursuit of any intellectual career from astronomy to necromancy. These were grammar, rhetoric and logic. In short, it insisted that its alumni could use their mother tongue, probably Latin, with the precision of a microtome and the accuracy of a vernier, could draw unchallengeable conclusions from incontestable axioms and defend the results before their peers and professors. The late eighteenth century (also slightly before my time) added the habit of patient and painstaking observation and a reliance more on life than learned literature, and defined the ideal embryo doctor.

For us there are many languages to learn. There are words we use among ourselves, the secret passwords to the craft, the mystery of medicine. It isn't only the hybrid classicisms like 'hypokalemia', two bits of Greek separated by a chemical symbol, or the ugly word 'contraindication'. Quite ordinary words take on a special meaning.

I still remember the scene at an Underground station in London one winter's night when a fellow student (and one who revels more in the pedantries of 'medispeak') asked a puzzled porter if 'the Tube was still patent'.

To us 'clinical' implies all that is imprecise, uncertain and ill-defined, but to the world outside it stands for cold, stark, impersonal attachment. Have you ever tried to convey to a layperson exactly what a lesion is? We know what we mean, but is it a malfunction or a misalignment? Only another medic knows.

There is another language too, the language of our patients, a thing of vernacular and euphemism, allusion and obsolete belief. How many lay words can you list for defecation or menstruation? What bizarre symptomatology (pointless, pompous word that it is) cannot a virus cause? What anxiety lies behind a reference to 'the old ticker'? There is a valid concern about the linguistic competence of some overseas graduates, but what examination paper can test that sort of English?

And, as if that were not enough, we have to interpret a silent language as well, of lowered eyes or twisting sweaty hands.

Where can we learn such things? Not from medical texts, not nowadays. The professional paper that described 'a remarkable feebleness of the heart's action', as Addison did in his classic description of the anaemia that bears his name, would seek publishers in vain. A psychiatric primer might shed some light, but one has first to translate the neologisms of that prolix trade. If we want to study the experts, those whose livelihood and fame depend on the shrewd observation of human behaviour, the telling sketch of human foibles, we must turn to the novelists and poets.

It was Dickens who described a desperate and successful struggle to bring a drowning rogue back to life. And who pointed to an odd and common paradox in most doctors, between respect for life however dim the spark and disgust for roguery however threatened with extinction. As their subject slowly responds to their efforts and resumes his unlovely self, so their interest wanes and they turn away from the man they have saved.

It was Thackeray who showed how a live philanderer becomes a dead hero on the battlefield. How a stray bullet converts a faithless, feckless husband into a deity to be worshipped by the wife he has betrayed.

It was Jane Austen who described the clear-eyed devotion of a daughter to a self-obsessed and neurotic father.

It's not surprising that so many of our number have turned the fragmented scraps of their patients' lives into coherent fiction. Somerset Maugham's notebooks show detailed accounts of what he witnessed of childbirth in the slums of Lambeth as a student 'on the district'. Keats reproduced the haunted hectic languor of active tuberculosis. Conan Doyle, scribbling between occasional consultations, drew thumbnail sketches of his characters with all the vivid accuracy ingrained by his medical training. An interest in words, their meaning and connections and the ideas that lie behind them, induced a paediatrician to write the standard reference for every journalist and author. Who sits down to write without *Roget's Thesaurus* at their elbow?

So let's choose our future colleagues from those who read beyond the set books of English studies; who occasionally desert the science curriculum to look into wider matters; who pry into Rabelais, that prince of bawdy physicians or Smollett, the surgeon's mate with a dirty mind but a brilliant pen; who wander the wide pastures of the library in search of what they want to know or ought to know about their fellows.

Let's look for those who know something of the lost art of precis, and can reduce the clotted prose of leader writers or columnists to a simple meaning, if meaning there be. Let's select those with a vocabulary large enough to encompass their ideas and understand other people's of whatever century. Let's recruit those who can express themselves with clarity, brevity and lucidity.

That's the kind of colleagues I'm looking for. People I can talk to, or better still, listen to. That way, there's a fair chance that the patients will be able to, too.

People who speak our language—as she is spoke.

my dear osbert

(A letter to a young colleague.)

Your mother, that charming woman, tells me that, after your latest brush with the examiners, you have decided to abandon your specialist career in favour of 'just' general practice. No doubt it is a disappointment to her. We will never alas hear her say, 'My son, the neurosurgeon', in that delightful throwaway voice of hers, but I hope you will find some compensation in this less glamorous pursuit.

Of course, you are luckier than I was. You have had the benefit of a Department of Community Medicine to lecture you on 'total care' and the 'team approach' and other more or less relevant topics. We only had lectures on public health (mostly drains and Acts of Parliament, I believe) from which we stayed away in droves.

I believe you were even taken to selected practices and heard about 'medicine in the community', as if it were different from anywhere else, and spent a week or two under some GP's roof, watching him write certificates, and chatting up his staff, or if you were lucky, his teenage daughters.

But I hope you will not take it amiss if I make one or two suggestions—not advice, one learns never to give that—which may ease your entry into this not inglorious pursuit.

You must prepare yourself for a new language, rich in imagery if imprecise in detail. Time is measured in 'a couple of'. This means more than one, rather than two, as you might think. As a prefix to 'years' it means within the last decade; to 'months', within a year or so; to 'weeks', some time this year; and to 'days', last pay day—or was it the one before? Severe pain 'touches you along a bit' or, in more desperate cases, 'warms' you. Severe stress, both physical and mental, may be such that your patient 'nearly goes out to it'. Happily, he or she usually returns.

You will be surprised to find that measles occurs in the newborn and recurs thereafter at monthly intervals during the first five years of life. It is accompanied by no systemic disturbance whatever and vanishes 10 minutes after the consultation. You will discover that most healthy children are brought to you only after an advisory committee of neighbours and paramedicals (hospital cleaners and elderly relatives of trainee nurses), chaired by one or other grandmother, has both diagnosed and outlined treatment. Your role is merely to confirm that the child is indeed 'cutting its teeth on the cross', has worms, or has 'outgrown its strength'. You would do well to comply with this role. You will talk yourself hoarse on the needless folly of circumcisions and then find yourself doing them.

You'll be invited to diagnose and avert pregnancy within hours, predict confinement to within minutes and prophesy death to the week, if not to the day. How I would like to meet one of those generous clairvoyants who 'only give someone six months to live'.

Wherever you settle, whatever colleagues you listen to, asthma is unusually prevalent. Indeed, an enterprising entrepreneur could make a fortune transporting asthmatics from the inland to the wheeze-free sea and taking their shore-dwelling fellow sufferers to the mountains on the return trip.

When you arrive in your chosen practice I would urge you as a first priority, after you have been looked over by the surgery staff and shaken hands with the local pharmacists, to find the machinery for dealing with the frankly mad. Inevitably, the first time you are on call alone someone will set about their nearest and dearest with a meat axe or vanish muttering into the loo with a shotgun. As it happens, the local psychiatrist will be on study leave, the essential paperwork will be locked in your partner's desk, and the only available major tranquilliser will look suspiciously out-of-date.

You arrive palpitating at the house to find a posse of police, a brace of cheerful ambulance officers and a swarm of distraught relatives. There is a cry of 'Here's the doctor now', and the crowd parts respectfully to watch the professional hero in action. You clutch your bag in self-defence—it's usually about the right height and weight for discouraging Alsatians, although Corgis can slip underneath and nip you—and you wonder what the hell to do. Should you stride boldly forward, faithful even unto death and address the sufferer with a few soothing words? But for one thing, your voice left with your remaining breath five minutes ago, and for another, what on earth do you say?

'Hello, 'ello, 'ello'? 'Good afternoon'? 'Put that bloody thing down'?

Or should you (and it will not surprise you to know that this is the course I favour) slip behind the largest available constable, say 'Alright lads, take him away' and stand by to treat major casualties?

Whatever you do, it's wise to cultivate your local police and ambulance officers. They've a lot going for them that you haven't, like bravery and experience. At my last major psychotic encounter, the sergeant and I documented, sedated and dispatched the patient before the bar of the club closed. We felt we'd earned a drink. So find out about the mental health procedures and laws first. You can join Rotary later.

In your first weeks in practice you may find yourself gratifyingly popular, particularly if you are young and single. This is a transitory placebo effect. Most of those who flock to you are suffering from curiosity or disenchantment with your colleagues. They will listen to you carefully, accept your diagnosis with respect, your treatment with gratitude and come back in a week or so unchanged. You will find yourself re-investigating your partner's clinical discards with gradually lessening enthusiasm, until you realise one day that what they're seeking is not cure but comfort. You are starting to become a GP.

You will have to accustom yourself to becoming a recognised and scrutinised member of the community. Your doings, your sayings, the very hairs on your face, are public property. A quite extraordinary number of local organisations will ask you out to dinner and make you lecture afterwards. The town snobs will make discreet investigations of your pedigree, the town drunks will conduct probing trials of your patience. You will pay for your standing with ectopic consultation, kerbside chats about grandma and nineteenth hole dermatology clinics and you will reap the rewards in soft fruits and hard liquor at Christmas time.

If you are wise you will give special care to plumbers, electricians and motor mechanics and bear with patience the demands of the small shopkeeper who tries to substitute tranquillisers for food and sleep and must always be seen at once.

The first sudden death after your arrival (don't be surprised if there's a run of them, it's not your fault) will spread widening ripples of consternation through your little world in the shape of mysterious chest pains and requests for ECGs from husky footballers in their late twenties.

Every time the Heart Foundation appears on television, or some professor has another beef about the pill, you will be driven mad with serum lipids and contraceptive conundrums. A hysterical newspaper headline will disrupt a score of successful therapeutic regimens. You will be weighed in the balance of *Woman's Day* and found wanting. No matter what your training, your experience or your ability, it can be discredited by any Brownie with a First Aid badge.

You will cajole and plead, threaten and implore the obese and watch them expand on starvation diets. You will inveigh against the evils of smoking and be given a hundred for Christmas. You will learn more about your patients from your receptionist (if she has been in the job for a long time) than from an hour-long interview; more about medicine from your local consultants, particularly if they are old enough to have been general practitioners themselves, than from the journals you no longer have time to read; more about drugs from the detailers than you are prepared to admit.

You will curse consultants who poach and bless the same men when they salvage your clinical disasters for you.

You will learn that the most important questions in practice are 'why', 'if' and 'when', rather than 'what' and 'how'. You'll find it maddening and fascinating, boring and exciting, stimulating and exhausting.

I think you'll like it.

euhemeroi

A nice word—its dictionary definition is 'the deification of dead heroes'. I don't know that I would rate my clinical heroes as gods—although some behaved like that—but heroes certainly. They are the ones whose aphorisms still ring through my mind during some clinical discussions.

'Gentleman', said one (a surgical knight who cut cabinet ministers if not kings in his heyday), 'gastric ulcers are like barmaids. Seldom as innocent as they appear. One must always take them out to be quite sure.'

They are the ones who still sit from time to time at my elbow along with my father, my patient's father and the other unseen players in the consultation.

You don't consciously select them, you don't even like some of them and you certainly don't know until long afterwards just how a phrase, an anecdote, a gesture, an attitude can shape your thinking or affect your outlook.

I would qualify the dictionary definition. Our heroes never die, unless increasing wisdom or bitter experience cause them, like old soldiers, to fade away. Who burns incense to a false god? But the others, the immortals, remain.

Who are my heroes? Top of the list I put my undergraduate tutors. It was an impressionable period of my life and it was they who first opened the door on a world so strange that I (who have moved in it for so long) have forgotten just how strange it is. From them I learnt the secret language, the signs and symbols of the Freemasonry of our craft. From them I acquired an immense and overweening pride in the power, the mystery and the mystique of medicine. I felt myself set apart, we all did, scornful of the other faculties and shunned by them in return. How we pitied and patronised the would-be lawyers, the embryo accountants, the fledgling engineers. They saw us as intolerably conceited snobs. And so we were.

There is an odd ambivalence in the medical student's attitude to their instructors. They are critical almost to the point of contempt, irreverent almost to the point of open insolence, and in a few months they ape them. They feel no shyness in disputing their conclusions or denigrating their skill when they can't recognise measles or put on a pair of surgical gloves in less than 20 minutes. We laughed at them when we should have wept for ourselves.

But the teachers had their revenge. Those clowns grew before our eyes to gods. We acquired their mannerisms, absorbed their prejudices and, it is to be hoped, gained some of their insight. The wise ones who introduced us to humility, the lofty ones who taught us dignity, the suave and flashy ones from whom we discovered guile, the hour-long analyst, the five-minute appendicectomist, the patient-sceptical obstetrician, the swift and brutal orthopod—they're all there somewhere at the back of my mind, murmuring, posturing, wielding a shining scalpel or shooting a gold-linked cuff.

Then as a swift antidote to all this meretricious glamour came real life—a good dose of it, too. I was an assistant beginning to doubt my omnipotence, watching my senior's calm solution of the problems I grappled with so noisily and ineffectively.

My first principal was slow of speech and unhurried of action. He put his facts together one by one, never moved until he knew exactly where to set his foot, accepted the vagaries of humanity with tolerance and gave opinions that all could follow and understand. He never sought to be liked; he never failed to be respected. I hope I shall never lose the influence of this wise midwife who brought a pathetic medical foetus big with book-learning and vanity into the real world of general practice. Like every other baby I bawled, but in time I walked and tried to match my infant stride to his.

I cut the chord and drifted off, met many other colleagues to watch and copy and many more patients to learn from and try to understand. Until I settled into the place that for the last 20 years and more I call my own. I found that some of the best teaching was available in the room next door and that the regard of a partner was more precious than the praise of a professor.

It was in the early years that the College invaded my little clinical world and admitted me to the company of what were said to be my peers, but I came to recognise as my betters. Perhaps that contact, that chance to see into the minds of better individuals, was the most valuable thing I bought with my subscription. It still gives me an immense and proper feeling of pride, on those rare occasions when I write the letters after my name, not that I am a Fellow, but that they are. At a sufficient distance I can claim professional kinship with Clifford Jungfer and Monty Kent Hughes, that I am in the same goodly company as Harvard Merrington, that I have sat at the same table (and many hours too) with Wes Fabb, Bill Jackson, David Watson and David Game. I could list so many more but it would be invidious to select among so many friends—and heroes.

There are the unseen heroes too: the stray lecturer who, in the midst of the dullest postgraduate lecture, lit a dark corner with a sudden lightning flash of explanation; the occasional journal writer who resolved a long-standing perplexity; the textbook that took me by the hand through some stressful situation. I have read Donald's *Practical Obstetric Problems* nearly as often as *The Pickwick Papers*, and that from a besotted Dickensian is praise indeed. I never understood general practice until I read Balint, never understood myself (or parts thereof) until I finished Berne's *Games People Play*.

Only now, when I find myself swapping experience and reminiscence with my trainee's knowledge and enthusiasm, do I realise what a strange ragbag is my medical education: a thing of shreds and patches, fading photographs and half-forgotten limericks. I still keep some of my ancient textbooks, yellowing memorials of green youth, marked by sweaty fingers, scored by underlined reminders, still faintly redolent of midnight oil. But when the last book is closed and carted to the tip, the last article torn up, the last journal thrown away, it's the people that remain: aphorisms, telling gestures, illuminating phrases and those who made them.

The teachers, the heroes, the Euhemeroi.

———————— being there

doctor in the wrong house ─────────────────────
it's all in the bag ─────────────────────────
gladys ──────────────────────────────────────
sick friends ────────────────────────────────
gotcha ──────────────────────────────────────
monday, bloody monday ───────────────────────
the doctor tells ────────────────────────────
my colleague from the congo ─────────────────
the copper bracelet ─────────────────────────
giving it away ──────────────────────────────
one eye on the cook ─────────────────────────
in at the death ─────────────────────────────

doctor in the wrong house

Early morning calls are always awkward, especially those that come between getting up and going to work. Do you sacrifice breakfast, or spend the rest of the day in vain pursuit of the hour lost at the beginning? This particular morning it came while I was in the shower, and I dripped my way tetchily to the telephone, dabbing here and there en route with an inadequate towel.

It was the hospital. With the maddening bonhomie of those who have been at work for a couple of hours already, Sister relayed the message. The individual concerned was not actually a patient of mine, but of Dr X, who lived 10 miles away. The son, passing his widowed mother's unit on the way to work, had observed that her emergency light was on and going inside had found her 'far from well'. He had relayed this comprehensive diagnosis to his wife, who had alerted the hospital, who had extracted me sketchily-dressed, drying like a shallow summer pond in sticky patches and 'far from happy'. Meanwhile, the dutiful son had switched off the warning light and sped on to an honest day's toil, no doubt heartened by the thought that his duty had been done.

The address? Oh well, I was told, it's one of the units on Main Street. Which narrowed it down to one of 25 scattered along the mile or so of our longest thoroughfare. Furthermore, Sister told me, it was unit two and she thought, only thought mind you, that it might be opposite the old garage that is now an antique shop.

Heartened by these useful clues I narrowed my search to the six units more or less opposite the former garage in question. The front door of unit two was open as confirmatory evidence of distress.

I barged in breezily, congratulating myself on a smart piece of detective work under trying circumstances. Perhaps my clinical acumen would be equally astute.

The front and the inner security screen doors swung to behind me, and I paused in the hall for sounds of life before announcing my healing presence.

Sounds there were: a pleasing light baritone mingled with steam and the sound of running water issued from what was patently the bathroom. It appeared that the hills were alive with the sound of something. It occurred to me that the lonely widow woman, however far from well, had some explaining to do. Unless she had taken in a pathologically insensitive lodger or—and here the realisation at last dawned—I was in the wrong house.

I turned to go. The screen door was solidly and unshakeably locked. I peeped hesitantly into the other rooms for means of escape. The windows were too small. There was no back door. I pondered my next move.

It seemed I had two options. One, I could poke my head cheerfully around the bathroom door and ask the way to the ailing lady, the nearest bus stop or indeed anywhere outside. Two, I could ambush the unsuspecting vocalist in his own hallway and hope to speak long and coherently enough to forestall the arrival of the police, fire brigade, ambulance officers, or any other agency he might enlist to eject his deranged and possibly dangerous intruder.

Happily, a final desperate inspection revealed that the door catch moved vertically not horizontally and I slunk out with skin and reputation intact. He will never know just how alive the hills were on that particular morning.

Thinking about it afterwards I wondered how the interview would have gone. I'm inclined to think that my explanations would have been accepted, especially with the corroborative evidence of my doctor's bag and its jumbled but essentially harmless contents.

Apart from that incident, I have twice in the past month broken and entered into a patient's home—once to talk to an immured depressive in the small hours and once at noon in search of an acutely dyspnoeic old gentleman who had vanished when the ambulance arrived. I felt neither guilt nor alarm on either occasion. For, together with the parson, we are about the only people likely to be excused for trespassing on a stranger's domain. We are, on the whole, benevolent burglars, credited with honourable intentions and harmless and unselfish motives.

The base of most of the criticisms of our calling is just that: we don't call any more. Behind those wistful laments for the 'good, old-fashioned family doctor' who was, in retrospect at any rate, tirelessly attentive and endlessly patient, if therapeutically impotent, is the just observation that we used to *call*, but now we send an ambulance or suggest a taxi. In isolating ourselves in shining surgeries, however deep the carpet, however smart the hardware, we reject the privilege of entering a patient's home, avoid the challenge of meeting someone on their own ground and thereby ignore the countless clues to character, outlook, adjustment and income that we all display at home. The rigid obsessive perfection of the migraine sufferer's front hedge, the drawn blinds of the depressive's living room, the cheerful squalor of the feckless, the pathetic decay of the neglected—it's all there for those who will go and see.

If you want to build or keep a practice, if you want to vanquish the alternative opposition or close the doors of the adjacent clinic, you should undertake home visits.

But do go to the right house.

——————————————— it's all in the bag

It was one of those mornings when you seem to be the victim of a global conspiracy of inanimate obstructions. I hadn't slept too well either and met the day with gritty eyes and second-hand skin.

It's not the hammer blows of fate that flatten us but the constant nagging taps of minor disaster. The butter is too hard, the toast too soft, the toaster won't pop and the paper won't unwrap. You set off determined to take cover from the inevitable malevolence of the day.

The hospital patient you have promised to examine in detail is striding about the corridor fully and irreversibly clad; the recovering hemi-paretic who is to walk for you today is rigidly blanket-bound; and the new diabetic for whom explanations and good counselling are due has taken permanent residence in the loo.

It was to be expected that my first consultation, a routine check-up, should turn up unsuspected lesions; that the 'just a repeat of the tablets doc.' should burst into tears at the door; that the X-ray developer needed replenishing again; and that the only Ventolin in the building was 12 months out-of-date. It was to be expected, was even reassuring, that the third telephone call of the morning should be from a so far unsuccessful suicide.

In a slurred and spasmodic voice she listed the awesome pharmaceutical cocktail she had swallowed yesterday lunchtime. Happily, none of the ingredients were prescription items and she appeared to have struck a judicious balance between stimulants and depressants that had left her puzzled vital centres with no option but to keep going. Her dominant mood appeared to be one of irritation. 'Why hasn't it worked?', she demanded peevishly.

I faced the familiar GP dilemma—leave a crowded surgery or defer a cry for help. Could I assume that nearly 12 hours after the event the conscious patient would remain so until I got there? I could scarcely tell her to ring me back if she went into a coma. So, like all my wise and experienced colleagues, I weighed the odds, brought my clinical judgment to bear, summoned years of hard-won experience to my aid and made an informed decision. In short, I took a punt.

'I'll be there at the end of the morning.'

I drew up at the house in due course, noticed with relief the absence of an ambulance, the police or peering neighbours, and reached into the boot with practised ease for my bag.

It wasn't there.

A less common problem now faced me—go back for the gear, or head into the house?

I felt extraordinarily naked walking up the garden path with no bag to swing, no badge of office, no staff of therapeutic comfort or wand of diagnostic magic. She had sent for me and, poor girl, that's all she got.

We sat on the edge of the bed and talked. As a concession to my status I took her pulse and tried to guess its volume, inspected her tongue and pupils but after that, it was just talk.

It was a pretty one-sided conversation. After a little verbal prodding she explained: a confused tale of an ex-husband who wouldn't leave her alone and a would-be husband who abruptly did just that; of errant children and uncomprehending parents. The sad cycles of betrayal and despair recurred from one generation to the next. The clear choices but impossible decisions, and then history repeated the same game of chess from checkmate to stalemate.

She told her story well: not without a wry self-deprecation, clear, somewhat detached, unsentimental and coherent. Between sips of milk for her ephedrine-parched tongue she outlined her reasons and detailed her activities. Her irritation at the failure of her plans was still directed at the means she had chosen—all that those carefully purchased and laboriously prepared medicaments had done was to make her sick. It simply wasn't good enough.

Psychiatric labels flitted through the back of my mind— schizoid, hysteria, masked depression? With a label I could act with certainty, without one there was only a question mark. I offered hospital refuge, psychiatric ward retreat, psychiatrists, psychologists and, as a last despairing resort, me (professionally, that is).

'Well, at least you could listen', she said with approval. I was not a shrink, 'but shouldn't you be seeing the real sick, not idiots like me?'

The time came for me to act. But how, without a bag to delve in or a prescription pad to scribble on? Worse still, the time had come for me to make a decision, to take another and perhaps final punt.

'No', she said, she wouldn't do it again, and then punctured my relief by adding, 'Not that way, anyway'.

'Yes', she said, she would come and talk to me again, or ask me to come if things were desperate, and with that we parted.

I went back to a late lunch and the security of my bag.

gladys

Just across the street from the back of the surgery, the entrance that we sneak into when we're late and sneak out of when we're lazy, is a flagpole and there most days flies a Union Jack, limp in the summer sun or straining bravely in the winter storms. There, alas, one recent day it drooped forlornly halfway down the pole. I checked the paper—despite an hour or two of oratory, the sovereign remained in regal health and the Ashes still remained where they rightfully belonged.

But the domiciliary nurse's car so often parked outside was not in sight, and then I realised: Gladys was dead.

One of the pleasures of living in a little town is the characters that give it personality and so many happy hours of conversation. One of the sadnesses of staying too long in a little town is seeing them go.

Where is Mrs M, whose angular uncompromising bicycle bisected impertinent traffic, a scarlet straw hat signalling her purposeful summer progress? Where is Danny, the happy imbecile, the uninvited voracious guest at every church fete or 'pleasant Sunday afternoon'? Where is the lady who extruded her lower dentures at every seventh breath until the nurses took them away from her and she pined away and died? Where is the bushman who haunted the police station with accusations of theft and mayhem? (He even accused me once of stealing his weekend meat.) Where are the felt-hatted sisters who sailed their ancient sedan disconcertingly around blind corners? Or the rich man who bought a new fridge to keep his chocolate in while he dug his garden in the sun?

Of this decaying Dickensian band, Gladys was a natural leader. Stomping on extravagantly concertinaed legs through the town, bowed with the wickedness of the world, leading every battle with her battered chin, she fought the good fight and neighbours fled at her approach.

She took on the ABC—something to do with children's television I think—and when that organisation broadcast *Play Group* regardless, enlisted the vicar to her cause. He, wise guileful shepherd that he was, referred her to the bishop and her ragged garden gained, temporarily, a purple stock. But his lordship's unction, his eloquent hands and silver tongue availed him not and he was numbered with the enemy.

Then she turned her attention to us. Weekly she ambushed an unsuspecting doctor in the car park and flattened him with a well-thumbed expose of the virtues of a quack cancer cure. Common courtesy demanded an appearance of attention, common cowardice an ambivalent endorsement.

One by one she pinned us down. The swift evaders, who smiled and fled, were bombarded with letters that ran through a predictable gamut from explanation to vilification. The courteously non-committed sooner or later confessed to scepticism and were later implicated in the great cancer conspiracy; and the rash unguarded opponents were fixed with her gimlet eye and publicly berated.

Then she got an SCC on one shin. To our credit, no one offered Laetrile from California or peach stones from the back yard (the nearest local substitute). To our surprise, she selected an orthodox colleague. To his surprise, she submitted gracefully to the fumbling inadequacies of standard treatment. And to everyone's astonishment, it worked.

With heroic magnanimity none of us said 'I told you so' and she forgave the profession for its lamentable success.

She turned her attention to other plots and scandals. Not, however, before a nasty threat to my partner of legal proceedings over his failure to diagnose another lesion on her shin at a consultation for a minor throat infection. He evidently compounded the offence by subsequently bidding her 'Good evening' and smiling—a clear case of wilful and deliberate negligence.

But she still came occasionally. She told the receptionist at 2 p.m. of her 2.15 appointment, reminded her at a quarter past and left untreated at 2.20.

Even her iron constitution eventually rusted. An inoperable bowel cancer put her to bed in the care of her two bachelor brothers and the calm and kindly supervision of the domiciliary nurses. Her limbs shrivelled and her abdomen swelled. The little wizened face fell in upon itself in a fuzz of whiskers.

She bore the indignities of dependence and the treachery of her failing body with the same spirit that raised the Union Jack daily in her garden.

But one day it only reached half-mast and she went off to corner some hapless angel about the inadequacy of her harp.

I often wondered what sort of wife she would have made to the man brave enough to take her on. Would she have subsided into orthodoxy and complacent conformity, or gained an ally in her zany crusades?

Would she have borne children, lithe tennis playing daughters and sturdy cricketing sons?

But she belonged only to her ancient brothers and the town that feared and cherished her for so long. And now it is a duller place.

Who now will raise the flag?

sick friends

'They ought to put them in the forces for a year or two, that would teach them.' Teach them what, I wonder? How to shine their toe caps or strip an M16? How to obey senseless orders without question, observe pointless petty regulations and pay respect where none is due? Some value in that I suppose, and more in learning the practical democracy of the barrack room, the art of evading authority, the science of scrounging and the shield of ignorance.

What did I get for enlisting? A baggy suit of blue-grey serge, a handful of brass insignia, six pairs of drawers (flannel), which I never wore and a pair of boots I never polished. ('What's the name of your batman, Sir? He's not turning you out properly.') I also earned a pair of ribbons for each shoulder, which entitled me to salutes from lesser breeds, but demanded a similar gesture in acknowledgment.

The weary flight sergeant charged with the impossible task of turning a dozen young doctors into officers, to say nothing of gentlemen, likened my salute to a chicken squinting down a telescope. They were masters, those men, of respectful denigration. Who else but a French head waiter can get so much genial contempt, devastating comment or cutting scorn into a single 'Sir'?

So what did I learn? I learnt my place and that's a vital lesson that all of us should learn sooner or later. I found out that there was a wider world than medicine and that my companions and masters valued me professionally (to some extent) as they valued the corporal who serviced the RT, the sergeant who ran the crash line, or the controller who did the talkdowns (a technician, useful, even essential, but not central to the scheme of things).

I learnt to live with my potential patients and to care for my actual friends. I became adept at fending off consultations in the ante room and examinations in the bar. I learnt, or tried to learn, the patterns of stress in the fit and confident—the run of trivial complaints, the rising bar bills, the falling tolerance—that worry, strain or simple fear could induce in the most dashing fighter pilot. I learnt, or tried to learn, at what stage to confront, when to talk to the CO and when to act on confidences hardly won or betray friendships freely given. And I learnt the price of failure—a shrivelled blackening limb protruding from a heap of smouldering aluminium, a laconic epitaph of 'pilot error' and an empty locker in the crew room. It made a tragic punctuation to the customary round of sweaty feet and snotty noses, injections and routine examinations, sanitary rounds and short arm inspections.

But I never learnt, and never have, the proper balance of personal concern and professional detachment that the care of friends involves. To see the man you fish with, work or play with at odds with his family and wonder when to intervene; to observe and recognise outside the usual setting the chest pain that might be angina, a belly ache that could be something more than last night's rum—is to question your own responsibilities.

It is all too easy to join the conspiracy of denial, or worse, get on the merry-go-round of fruitless investigation and pointless treatment. It is too tempting to overlook or overtreat your friends.

Time and disaster have humbled the brash young medical officer of more than 30 years ago. I have learnt to qualify my certainties, temper my enthusiasms and mute my prophecies. I know, if nothing else, that nothing is ever quite so bad or so good as it seems at first and that the cost of my mistakes is borne by others, though the memories of them are my alone.

When a friend is sick you cannot but search within yourself for signs of failure or delay. You cannot but share the dismay and irrational anger of one challenged by life itself. You cannot avoid unreasonable hopes or unjustifiable dread. You too, look wistfully to the past and fearfully to the future.

So, my friend, as you set off to the alien world of medical technology, disabled, anxious and finally alone among strangers, you carry with you, among the lab reports and X-ray pictures packed with your pyjamas and paperbacks, my care, not unmixed with regret, my concern, not only for yourself and our friendship. I shall look for your return so that we may both begin the business of re-adaptation to an altered life from a continuing trust.

In my service days, the final chilling column in any medical report was headed 'disposal'.

I look forward to writing the usual comment, 'Medicine and duty', for both of us.

gotcha

There is a magic indefinable point in any enduring relationship when, by some subtle chemistry, the whole thing changes. The mixture becomes a compound, the solution throws down one reluctant crystal and then a coloured cloud of something new and indissoluble.

It's like that in medicine. You and the patient have met a dozen times or more, have exchanged courtesies and, to a limited extent, confidences. Then one day, for no apparent reason, the tenuous bond solidifies. For the first time you see each other as individuals and glimpse behind the outer walls at something of the inner chambers of each other's lives.

'Now', says the patient, 'I can really tell you.'

'Now', you say, 'you will really listen.'

It's a strange, illuminating, even slightly threatening moment, when you exchange vulnerabilities and deal with each other face-to-face. You are awarded a licence to explore, but will pay for it with the same coinage. It's fascinating to mark the point at which it comes, tantalising to guess what circumstance has brought it about.

In the UK, where patient and doctor are bound by administrative concurrence, it's less easy to separate. There are forms to fill in and letters to write before moving on. Patient and doctor are more likely to tolerate minor personal disharmonies, to wait for some definite offence before finally sundering the official connection. It was there that I learnt that one of the solid foundations to a doctor–patient relationship could be a good row. Some unjustified irritation on my part, unwarranted assumption on his or hers, would explode a trail of gunpowder that had trickled unremarked between us for months.

It was as if, after weeks of ducking and weaving, sparring and shadow boxing, we came to grips at last and discovered what we expected of each other. The air cleared, we were finally free to bargain, adjust and move on to more fruitful purposes. Once I dropped the maddening mask of cool, overly-courteous equanimity and he or she the tedious shield of unappeasable complaint, there were good things to be done together.

If they were done well you achieved the ultimate accolade of 'My own doctor', against whom others were measured and found wanting. You were the one invited to sit in judgment on the opinions of all the rest, however erudite or honoured. With the subtle syntax of possession, the patient moved from being 'a patient of mine' to 'my patient'.

I often think that half the tensions between the specialists and ourselves arise from that latter phrase. When you hear an obstetrician describe someone you have referred as 'my patient', it's hard to ignore a jealous protest from within. 'But she's mine', you say to yourself. 'I sent her and I'll take her back.' And while we bicker over the body, she very properly wanders off to less possessive advisers.

Because, of course, in the end, we do not own each other, however strong the bond may be. We lend and borrow only for a while. Everybody keeps something back, guards some inviolable corner against all intruders, we no less than others. If you would carry a light into another's mind, it must shine no less brightly upon your own.

Where there is freedom of choice and wide choice, as there is these days, it seems to take much longer to reach a point of trust. The patients search for some ideal abstraction—instantly, exclusively available, tirelessly compliant, knowing what is wanted without inquiry, giving it without demur. We, for our part, seek another myth—fluent, rational, responsive and grateful.

No wonder neither party is content.

'Trust me', you say.

'Show me', the patient says. And there is a disgruntled silence.

And every now and then (and, so help me, I don't know why) it isn't like that at all.

We all have patients that we cannot like. We are all aware of those who dislike us, but still return. It isn't skill. We all have patients whose belief has been betrayed, whom for one reason or other have just cause for reproach.

It isn't similarity of temperament or equality of social standing—in fact, it is often the reverse. There is respect in it and understanding. Perhaps the closest word is regard. You look at each other with unclouded eyes and accept the weaknesses and braveries, the honesties and evasions, without criticism. You appreciate one another—and that too has another meaning, for to appreciate is to grow in value.

And one fine day it comes together and there is one patient for whom you are always on call, but who never abuses that unspoken privilege. You catch unawares a tone of voice. You intercept a glance and you both say under your breath, 'Gotcha'.

monday, bloody monday

I knew it was going to be a hard day. There are Mondays when, if I don't exactly spring out of bed, I slide almost willingly to part the drawn curtains, spot the newspaper on or adjacent to the drive below and amble readily enough to the shower, muesli for breakfast and into the street with scarcely a backward glance at the squandered leisure of the last weekend.

There are other awful mornings when the luxury of lying in, so unattainable in vacation time, seals the eyelids, glues the body to the bed and tunes the ears reluctantly to the weary jocularities of morning radio. It is on such days when those who telephone demand a visit and those who don't expect one; when annual check-ups drop in without warning; pensioners drag driving licence applications from their pockets; and would-be pensioners bring in two-page interrogatories from the Department; when the normally brief become discursive; the usually stoic, tearful; and the dwindling stock of equanimity is exhausted by 11 o'clock; and you pick up the very last record of the very last—praise God—patient and find beneath it a visiting card.

The reps are in town.

You sweep your eye around a miraculously empty waiting room and there, lurking immersed in last year's *Woman's Day*, briefcase neatly parked beside far too shiny shoes, they wait in ambush.

Wait, poor devils, and wait and wait. Impelled by a distant and menacing sales manager, inured to insult, accustomed to snubs, unable to answer back, no less hungry than the target and no less anxious for release, they wait on your capricious pleasure. Here, at last, after the long morning is a legitimate Aunt Sally to be interrupted, hectored and derided, whose only defence is respectful deference, unsoundly based, and propitiatory gifts of ballpoint pens.

Sometimes, perhaps for protection, they come in pairs and the one you vaguely know brings along a stranger, suaver still and faintly menacing, who watches his or her protege watch you. I rather enjoy these encounters, diverting my ticklish questions and polite, I hope, derision to the intruder, while the underling perceptibly relaxes.

Sometimes we the customers listen in pairs, one seated at the desk, one sprawled across the corner, quizzing the hapless advocate for yet another non-steroidal anti-inflammatory, but grabbing the largesse.

And sometimes, more and more it seems, the rep is female. The companies with a shrewd and complimentary perception of the innate chivalry of masculine practitioners entrust their message to young women, at whom we gaze with undisguised awe, while a polished expose floats unheeded across the desk. We accept the sticky notepads with servile gratitude and fill our shelves with packaged samples that alas last longer than the fading aura of expensive perfume that wafted them to us.

'Have you any questions, doctor?', asked one of a colleague of mine.

'As a matter of fact yes', he said. 'Are you free for lunch?'

And she was. They were last heard of in Beijing I believe, where reps are rare and female reps unknown.

The drug companies, those multinational brigands who hold the sick to ransom, or so the papers say, show a kindly face to us their customers, or is it their agents? The young man dealing yet another ace from the overloaded deck of Blankoprils listens respectfully to one dotard's impression of one unusual case. He makes us feel that Merck will take note, Sharpes' enthusiasm will be blunted and Dohm will become a dome of silence, in the face of one country doctor's unscientific prejudice.

They never say, as well they might, that without the effort, the expertise, the painstaking research, the blind alleys so expensively explored, we would still be treating syphilis with arsenic, pneumonia with oxygen, mania with bromides, and cancer with sympathy and nothing else. That it was phenothiazines that unlocked the doors of the asylum, streptomycin that emptied the sanatoria.

Instead, they send their emissaries to flatter and explain in so many guises. There are the old stagers who greet you with the cheering news that they have nothing new this week, who chat and leave their needed samples sure of their welcome, but never outstaying it, who mute the brazen trumpets of the marketing machine to persuasive whispers and who are as tried and trusted as the drugs they sell. There are those who without positive disloyalty to the company that hires them somehow communicate a welcome tinge of scepticism, who ring the familiar changes—newer, safer, stronger, cheaper, easier to take—with a lurking glimmer of disbelief.

Have we been bribed? I doubt it. I like to think that my price is higher than a calendar, a raffle ticket for a stethoscope, or a dinner at a local pub. One biro is very like another, one pub supper like most of those—Blankoprils has much the same effect. Most of the specialists imported by a company to push a product are at pains to be objective, even critical—if not to bite, at least to nibble the hand that feeds them and their audience.

I have accepted gifts, expensive medication gratis for a needy patient; have had casual queries exhaustively pursued and information tediously extracted; all without cost or apparent obligation. I do not look to them for knowledge, but I sometimes gain it. I do not earn their courtesy, but it seldom fails. I may show scant consideration, but I am usually given it.

Even those others, the too eager, the too glib, the too anxious to press a sweaty palm into yours, the ones who raise the hackles and set you shifting uneasily in your seat, have their uses at the end of a hard morning—especially on Monday, bloody Monday.

the doctor tells

'Whoever would lie usefully should lie seldom' (Lord Hervey).

A little after Christmas this year I was visiting a patient of mine (and previously of my late partner). She had an inoperable breast cancer, a horrible, hard ulcerating mass, which she had borne without complaint or definitive treatment for something like 10 years. She and her sister lived with her married daughter and family and the lesion first came to light during her sister's final illness. For that reason and perhaps a personal dislike of fuss, to say nothing of the additional burden on an already stressed household, she said nothing of it.

As a human being, I could not but admire the uncomplaining fortitude with which she endured what could not be cured. As a doctor, of course, I found it all quite intolerable. With that officious solicitude with which we invade other people's lives uninvited I found myself uttering that awful phrase that I dread to hear: 'Something must be done.'

We had a long and largely amicable argument. Did her people know? No. Isn't it about time they were told? Why? We went through it step by step and I struggled with a self-righteous indignation. To any doctor, the only thing worse than a patient who won't get better is one who will not even let you try to help them get better. Finally, she played her ace. How could she tell them after all this time? Let me do it, I offered. Then to my astonishment and, I must add chagrin, she surrendered. Alright then, you do it. When? Now.

I mentally abandoned my first two appointments already due at the surgery and went in search of daughter and son-in-law. And while I opened doors, called and at length found them, I asked myself how the hell I'd got into this. They came, puzzled and concerned. I cleared my throat.

'Do you know what's wrong with your mother?'

'I think so.'

'What?'

'Well, it's the word we don't use.'

With brusque persistence better suited to those inquiries where people are invited to help the police, I finally elicited the dreaded word.

As you doubtless have already guessed, they knew what she knew, but she didn't know that they knew. For all the gravity of this revelation there were strong elements of farce in the whole situation and I left shamefaced, wondering not for the first time in my career just what I had achieved.

I think, on reflection, that it was probably worthwhile. It must have made conversation a bit easier in that household and it certainly paved the way for more positive palliation. But it raised other questions too.

We tend to think that the move towards exposure is a new idea, that only our bright and fearless generation can say 'cancer' aloud, uninflected by fear or pity. But there was a Royal Cancer Hospital in my young days—until they changed the name to the Royal Marsden. We take pride in our growing recognition of death as a certainty to be planned and cared for—and have founded special places to do it in. A generation ago, they called them 'homes for the dying'. That's plain enough. This coy disregard for reality is relatively new and, thank heavens, is already fading away. The moral must be then, as this family found out, that it's always better to tell the truth.

But is it? About a month ago, another patient reported what sounded like a Transient Ischaemic Attack while he was away on holiday. By the time he reached me he had no signs and was only too ready to accept that adding half an aspirin to his effective hypotensive regimen was probably all that was necessary. Until, a few days later, he had another attack, this time with signs for all to see for a day at least and a transient and uncertain carotid murmur.

The radiologist rang me. He had suffered not one but two small cerebral haemorrhages, one on each side. The patient was still with him, relaxed, cheerful and apparently unimpaired. Which was more than could be said for the radiologist, who asked rather querulously what was to be done with my patient. He didn't add, 'Get him out of here', but the message was clear.

It was, of course, Friday afternoon; the neurologist, naturally, was on holiday in New Zealand; of the two locally available physicians one, obviously, was away for the weekend and the other, inevitably, had a previous commitment and wouldn't be here until Monday. I took a deep breath, 'Send him home and I'll go round and see him and [blessed phrase] sort something out'. Off I went to assess, explain and make some sort of plan. He greeted me cheerfully. 'Tell me it's nothing serious', he said. 'You can lie to me if you like.'

Was that attitude so very wrong? I could indeed have lied to him, taken refuge in comforting, meaningless labels such as 'turns', 'spasms', 'congestion' and 'little clots'. Or I could have sat down and scared the pants off him with an exhaustive list of daunting diagnostic possibilities, beginning with cerebral tumours and ending with bleeding disorders and probably a blood pressure high enough to ping any vessel.

What I did do was tell him some of the truth. 'You've had two little bleeds into the brain [true—I even knew the dimensions, thanks to the radiologist]. They've stopped now [I think they have, but how can anybody tell?]. I don't know exactly why [true indeed] and it will have to be looked into next week [true, if nothing catastrophic happens sooner]. In the mean time, you can go into hospital [which gets me off the hook, but may sidetrack you] or I can watch you at home.' Which is what I eventually did. The next week I handed him, still cheerful, to the neurologist. Investigations are, as they say, still proceeding.

Now, pondering that episode—not the management, it was either wise or foolhardy, no one can settle that—I wonder whether the patient has the right to ask to be lied to and the doctor a duty to comply? In this case it was explicit and perhaps facetious. Would I have been remiss to take him at his word or heartless not to? In other, most other, cases it is implicit. 'Tell me the truth, doc., I can take it' often reads 'Tell me the truth if you think I can take it', and since I don't know what experience or resources they may have I can't tell. In still other cases, the majority I suspect, it's the relatives who ask 'Don't tell him, doc., it'll kill him'. Sometimes maybe it does—so too does the disease you are not allowed to name. If a patient asks you to tell them outright, of course, you must and run the risk of setting up the very situation I described earlier.

I have to my shame co-operated in deception. Some years ago the husband of a woman with a literally open-and-shut case of pancreatic cancer begged me not to tell her. He said it would kill her. It hasn't yet, but his aortic aneurism burst a couple of year's later—and they both knew about that. Was the husband wrong? Or the histologist? Or has she known all along?

I'd love to ask her one day. I wonder if she'd tell me the truth.

my colleague from the congo

From time to time, when the press perversely misinterprets our behaviour and an ill-directed spotlight casts a greedy shadow behind our well-intentioned profile, we start to worry about our image. Mostly, it takes the form of unpublicised protests about the media, sometimes it engenders letters to the Journal—all honest explanation and righteous indignation—and less often, there is a call for a counterblast and our subscriptions are diverted to the pockets of a public relations expert. It's called PR for short and we all know what that means.

There are dinners at our expense and media releases, sometimes even a truncated interview on television, when a forthright colleague comes over as shifty and evasive and reveals that the cares of office have thinned his hair and lined his face. We tell our spouses what he should have said and it all settles down again.

The patients still present themselves at the surgery; the often-predicted demise of general practice is postponed; and the image is put back in the cupboard a little dustier, a little less recognisable.

My own characteristically ambivalent attitude to the press is coloured by family connections. I admit to a journalist son, another son who is a public servant and a daughter with a lively interest in alternative medicine. Prejudice, it seems, is not genetically determined.

So I know something of the other side of the newspaper world and the outlook of those men and women who, like us, are publicly castigated and privately consulted every day of their working lives.

Similarly, I have heard of public servants trying to negotiate with greedy self-seekers on twice their income and less than half their principles. Nor do I need to be told about my manifest deficiencies that drive the gullible to ginseng or iridology.

The journalist came home a month or two ago after an extended African tour that ended in a bedsitter in Golders Green (that long-established clearing in the jungles of North London). He brought us presents. Mine, in fact, was more of a presence. It was a life-sized mask, carved from some jungle wood, bedaubed with coloured clay eyebrows, befringed with a coarse straw beard and bedecked with half a dozen cows teeth in a cheerfully upturned mouth. My son said it reminded him of me. He's old enough and big enough to get away with that sort of thing these days.

You know, he was right. Perhaps a little unkind in the cosmetic features—my teeth are not that white any more—but in its essentials a true and proper likeness.

Each day, as I look at it on the consulting room wall, it confirms my belief that in our separate ways we ply the same trade and share the same problems. Doubtless there are cultural differences, but I swear that as I usher in some exasperating valetudinarian and catch sight at my Congo colleague, he winks at me.

'I get them too', he seems to say. 'Will they take the mango juice three times daily as directed by the medicine man? Will they hell! As like as not they'll creep off to the missionaries and waste good money on antibiotics or some other rubbish.

'Bad debts? You're telling me nothing. I had to give up putting spells on slow payers, I was losing too many customers. Just as you're settling down to some real medicine—a nice diabolic possession say or someone who's turning into a goat—some bureaucrat from the chief's office is on the drums; rhinoceros horn is now an authority item, for heaven's sake.

'Then some old bludger who claims he was trodden on by an elephant in the Matabele Wars wants a bigger pension. You know the kind—never satisfied until they've got a free hut and as much tax-free tapioca as they want. Never seen a spear thrown in anger most of them.'

I return to my day's work, comforted that I'm not uniquely selected to suffer the tribulations of the trade; that all over the world, doctors of one kind or another are putting on white coats or yellow ochre, waving wands or stethoscopes, chanting their various spells, prescribing their various nostrums, trained by their common experience and distinguished by their particular beliefs. Above all we share that uplifting conviction that we alone are right. Our science is the true science and theirs, whoever they are, is mere mumbo jumbo.

In most infections we, the Westerners, had the edge until AIDS came out of Africa and scared us into re-learning the lesson that hygiene is the cure. Only this time it's sexual hygiene.

In the wilderness between pathology and witchcraft I wonder if my mate from the Congo is not in front. In those ill-charted seas where sadness has physical signs and illness spiritual effects, what is needed is not patience or tranquillisers, empathy or surgery, but magic.

'Make me better', they say. But how? What's the cure for a drunken husband, a feckless youth, a rotten job, or no job at all?

Our society, I grant you, might jib at some Congolese solutions. A discreet dose of Cobra venom intradermally administered or a brisk exhibition of rawhide externally applied would upset us just as much as they might find it cruel to shut away their elders in geriatric ghettos or offer nothing to the woman who stays at home to care for the family while other mothers go to work.

Both societies throw up interlocking personal problems that to the eye of science are insoluble and to the feelings of humanity are heartrending. Both yield only to hope—and magic.

So from now on, I shall no longer excuse my occasional absences from the surgery by admitting to taking a holiday.

'What again?' is the common aggrieved rejoinder.

No, I shall simply say I was taking a spell.

──────────────────────────── the copper bracelet

Not long after I returned from fishing (yes I did, thank you), in that relaxed but meticulous post-vacation frame of mind, when we listen and look and present a jovial imperturbable face to all that come, a man came in to my surgery.

He was in late middle age—well older than me anyway—and beginning to suffer the urinary embarrassments of that time of life. He was a retired engineer, a self-labelled, self-made man who perhaps should have called in a sub-contractor for the plumbing. He demanded and got as full an explanation of the anatomy, physiology, surgery and therapeutics as I could furnish without a book in front of me. I drew pictures and offered rather rubbery statistics. I touched lightly enough on the possible mishaps and heavily enough upon their rarity to encourage him and vindicate me should anything go wrong. I discussed his other health problems—the manifest obesity, the borderline hypertension—and sketched out for him the profile of the perfect anaesthetic subject.

He was wary rather than suspicious, penetrating rather than sceptical and somehow treated me as an instructed but fallible technician who had to make out a case in terms that were both rational and convincing. Which was probably about right.

He did not, I'm happy to say, demand surgery without complications, procedures without discomfort, or drugs without side effects. But he did look for the sort of mechanical certainty, degrees of tolerance and certainties of outcome that belong more properly to his craft of engineering than to my imperfect and hazardous art.

He did not, I was delighted to find, assume that a general practitioner is by definition too lazy to find out the latest techniques so fully documented in women's magazines, too ignorant to be aware of the perils of drugs so freely debated in the daily newspapers and too obstinate to listen to objections soundly based on the reported wisdom of the hairdresser, the cleaner and the neighbourhood iridologist.

'It won't do me any harm, will it?', asks another doubtful patient, baulking at the proffered prescription. And yet again I repress the reply I long to give, 'As a matter of fact, it will probably kill you. That's why I chose it'.

'My beauty consultant says this could thin my skin', remarks a supercilious patient reading my prescription. And again I whisper internally, 'Madam, nothing short of a belt sander could do that'.

What other profession is so frequently contradicted by the amateur? The voice of the accountant is the voice of doom—until the demand comes in. The word of the lawyer, if you can afford it, is the voice of God. I assume as I climb into a Boeing plane that the designers have got it right. I rely without hesitation on the durability of lift cables, the stability of skyscrapers and the buoyancy of ferry boats. If the jeweller tells me my watch needs cleaning I acquiesce without question, even though another jeweller in the adjacent street said and did the same thing the week before.

I can only think of the fictional police detectives who suffer as we do. Who through each succeeding chapter are denigrated and humiliated by the amateur. They, like us, are assumed to be dull, vacuous and stupid. They, like us, act as a sort of lay figure, a little light relief in the pursuit of villainy or health, a wooden target for Mr Punch's baton. If Sherlock Holmes is ever found murdered, garrotted perhaps with a violin string or beaten to death with a magnifying glass, don't arrest Professor Moriarty, the Napoleon of crime. Concentrate your inquiries on Inspector Lestrade—or Dr Watson.

Back to my interrogator. He had the grace to apologise for his persistence. It was, he explained, a simple problem in mechanics to him, a loose valve to be re-ground, a doubtful washer to be replaced. While he did not doubt my competence, he had to understand both the problem and the solution. He believed, very properly, in taking nothing on trust. I was neither a father nor an uncle to him—an elder brother perhaps, but certainly not an idiot cousin.

At last, it was my turn. 'May I ask you a question?'

'Fire away, doc.'

'Why do you wear that copper bracelet?'

giving it away

A couple of years ago a young man limped into the surgery and, as I followed him down the corridor to my room, presented his diagnosis. He had 'done his back'.

It was a familiar story and a familiar picture. Two men carrying a heavy object, one slips and the other twists and does his back. It was a familiar and depressing situation: a strong, healthy breadwinner battling unaccustomed pain and even more unusual immobility. After a week or two it would get better, the local tenderness would subside and apart from some morning stiffness and a tendency to get stuck in armchairs, there would be a comforting anticipation of normality again. Next week or the week after it would be back to work, but just be careful how you lift.

But it wasn't in this case. The straight leg raising started to diminish, the doubtful ankle jerk disappeared altogether and we were both looking at months of enforced idleness, sceptical employers, conflicting opinions, reports, recriminations and despair. Doctor and patient, employee and employer, would exchange barrages from the trenches dug by the lawyers and the case become a cause.

You, the doctor, vainly patrol the wilderness of cure or settlement, heading off, if you can, injudicious surgery, the fatuous advice of sympathetic onlookers and ill-considered resort to expensive alternatives. From the security of your position and the reasonable certainty of your income, you prescribe rest and change the analgesics, issue certificates and counsel patience to a once-fit young man imprisoned in his own home for an indefinite term, unable even to mow the lawn.

In this particular instance we went through the long, frustrating progression from hope to anger to apathy, until at last it was settled and he vanished. There were no more reports, no more certificates and I assumed he was back at work—or written off.

Then, one day he reappeared. He was brisk, rather overweight and rather overbearing, as are most of those who run their own business. The man who for a long time had come so often that it was an unspoken reproach, who depended on me for reassurance I could not give and went away with tablets I did not want to give, now saw me as a tiresome but necessary distraction in a busy day. In fact, much the same as I feel about the dentist.

He wanted a thorough check-up and that, within my limitations, he got. At last, while he was dressing and admitting ruefully to his need of exercise and moderation I asked, 'What about your back?'

'Oh', he said, 'I've given that away'.

He told me the story. In the long-enforced immobility of his injury he had put himself through a course in business management. It had become obvious to him that he would never again earn his living by physical effort, so when a settlement was offered he grabbed it. Despite the urging of his lawyer, who doubtless could—eventually—have got him more and cost him more, he used this money to change his life. He started an agency. I didn't follow the details, but it involved promotion work in the sporting world and many hours driving and flying interstate. Like all self-employed people he hovered between too much work, which was overwhelming and too little, which was alarming and if the shape of his stomach and the diameter of his neck was anything to go by, he was thriving

'But what about your back?' I asked.

'It's still a bastard. Some days it takes me 10 minutes to get out of the car after a long trip and I still have to sleep on the floor some nights, but I don't think about it.'

Since then, I have spent a lot of time pondering the moral of this story. It confirms a long-held suspicion that an illness can be a disaster or an opportunity. Nobody must or should proceed inevitably down one avenue. There are other routes to the goal, or perhaps other goals. For some, death is just a shortcut. A period of rest and reflection is a necessary pause in any life. Every advance should include an occasional retreat. I am not advocating prolapsed discs as a path to grace, still less that any kind of pain is the way to paradise. The cure for toothache is codeine, not little homilies on the nobility of suffering. I suspect that, on the whole, suffering ennobles only those who were noble to start with.

As Dr Johnson said, 'Disease produces much selfishness. A man in pain is looking after ease. It is so very difficult for a sick man not to be a scoundrel.' But that opens a whole new debate. Our job, after all, is to offer ease, if ease there can be and suspend any sort of judgment about scoundrelism. If Keats, the immortal apothecary, wrote immortal verse because he was tuberculous—which I doubt—this very mortal apothecary would prefer rifampicin.

But what my ex-patient suggested to me was something different. If we are to survive physically and mentally we should, in fact must, accept disease or disability for what it is—an accident. If the physician can palliate our symptoms to the point that we can concentrate on other things and provide the ease that we are looking for, then there is a chance to take stock, to fill the vacant spaces of our mind with new material, to search in other directions for a path to follow. We can acquire a fresh direction and, in the process, give our back away.

one eye on the cook
and the other up the chimney.

I admit that I find squints unnerving. There is the recurring difficulty of deciding which eye to look at, the temptation to look away and the embarrassment of concentrating my empathetic gaze on an organ that abruptly shifts and almost disappears, while its fellow watches with wry amusement. If I pick the right eye it is almost impossible not to steal an occasional glance at the antics of the other and be caught doing it.

Those unfortunates in whom the squint is convergent carry with them an air of introspection that makes me feel that I am intruding on some momentous internal debate, but those with the divergent variety are even more unsettling to me.

So I was never entirely at ease with the lady who first came to me a few years ago, resigned to her angina, faintly irritated by her recurrent urinary infections and classing them with her demanding and insensitive husband as among those things that must be endured since none, it seemed, could be permanently cured.

She was, in her gentle, kindly way, an arch manipulator. She soon trained me to repeat the tablets when required, to prescribe the antibiotics when *she* felt they were needed and to give the preferred hypnotic without sage advice about drug-free slumber. I tried, of course, to be a good GP. I allowed her to suffer the discomfort of dysuria, the social penalties of frequency until the urine culture came back—usually negative. But in the end I succumbed and felt embarrassed by her gratitude.

I saw her through a prolonged ischaemic episode and all the subsequent investigations and I accepted that cardiac surgery was not for her. As we got to know and trust each other better she told me a little of her home life and I was not surprised when she decided she would endure no more and abruptly decamped. She found a little flat with a large garden only a couple of streets away where, after 30 years or more of matrimony, she hoisted the flag of independence.

Then the cordite fumes of Tobruk supplemented by 40 years of 40 cigarettes a day caught up with her husband and unhesitatingly she went back to nurse him.

I didn't look after him, but I did try to support her through days and nights of constant attendance on a difficult man, dying the slow dreadful death of failing breath. I tried to prepare her for the inevitable collapse after the inevitable outcome.

It came, of course. Sorrow beyond the reach of tranquillisers, guilt, regret and misery. She did not weep—in my presence at any rate—she did not repine or reminisce, except perhaps in her violent dreams. She just withdrew.

I gave her antidepressants—and took away the tranquillisers. She said she was better, but her aching eyes denied it. I learnt from her that a morning appointment meant misery for both of us, but afternoons offered hope. I suggested psychiatrists, but it was always 'not now' or 'not yet' and I acquiesced.

Then one day, after a particularly fruitless session, after I had pushed the antidepressant level to what the experts deem therapeutic—and the GPs toxic—and absolutely nothing had changed, I declined to be manipulated any more.

This woman was beyond me. She was clinically depressed and although still functioning, her self-imposed retreat would sooner or later become a rout and I would have to answer to myself for the consequences.

I put the hard word on her. She was sick and I had signally failed to help. It was time—long past time—for a fresh approach, a better expert, more practised management. She stalled, of course, but for once I stood my ground and perhaps because of the trust account we had deposited between us over the years, she eventually agreed. 'But not 'now, let's wait another week': I wouldn't. The appointment was made, a daughter enlisted as escort and I waited for her to collect the long, long letter of referral.

Then she appeared unannounced one morning. For the first time in our association she was smartly dressed, discreetly made up, positively cheerful. She was, and she said it with conviction, so much better. She'd been out to this morning tea, that evening party, had bought a new wardrobe, visited a fresh hairdresser and was sleeping like a baby.

I took a bit of convincing, but I knew she was right and the benevolent spy network of a little town confirmed it.

What had happened? Had that unconscionable mass of medication finally caught up with her? Had the hours of circular discussion finally found a tangent? Was the threat of psychiatry more shocking than the ECT that she might have been prescribed? Was it God, or glands, or common sense?

I too was grateful, but I didn't know whom to thank and I was faintly but definitely annoyed. How dare she get better without my sanction? When with all the weight of my knowledge, depth of my experience, breadth of my skill, I had told her she needed even greater expertise. I was really quite upset with her.

Or was it those eyes?

in at the death

Some names penetrate the barriers we build around our leisure. For some patients, we are always on call—the dying, the soon to be born, the personal friends who are patients and the patients who have become personal friends. The list is short and ever-changing and creates problems for our minders—if we are lucky enough to have them.

The call that came through just as I was leaving for surgery was for a name that had been on this list for a long time. It was about him, but not from him. His sister had found his front door open, his bedroom door closed and a radio playing within, but no answer to her call.

'I didn't like to go in', she said, 'not on my own'.

It was enough to tell me what she half-guessed and I half-dreaded.

We were both right. I will spare you the details. It was the act, not the method, that shocked; the decision, so deliberate and irrevocable that stunned us both.

The first moves were simple, but not easy. I had to confirm what we both already knew, break the news that would shock but not surprise, search in vain for some adequate consolatory phrase, find and put the kettle on for tea—that indispensable anodyne of catastrophe—and settle to the telephone. A policewoman with exactly the right mix of solicitude and efficiency came and set the legal wheels in motion. I left to gather up the threads of a morning's work and later, when activity gave way to reflection, I reviewed the victim's life as I had known and played a part in it and wondered what I or others could have done to recognise and reverse a decision so deliberately executed.

There was no real reason to ask why he had done it. It was not a case of 'the balance of his mind being disturbed' as coroner's juries once quaintly said. Rather, it was the reverse. For the first time in many years his mind was settled—with tragic finality. There was no facile psycho-pathological label to be attached, no scientifically-authenticated physical disorder, though there were elements in plenty of both. There was no social or economic disaster looming, though he had surmounted plenty of these in his time. His simple wants were well if not extravagantly catered for and a concerned and loving family were as close to him as he would allow. He was alone by choice.

Why then?

Let me tell you what I knew of him. I met him first as a rather tiresome casualty who presented late and quite often, with renal colic and a humble and gentle persistence that usually won him pethidine. 'Aha', you say, 'just what I'd expect, a druggie'.

But he wasn't. He did have renal stones, showers of them, and the combined resources of two professorial units and three (I think) urologists confirmed the fact, and could only suggest less milk, more water and, by implication, pethidine as before.

I got to know him during this time and learnt something of his childhood on the family farm—of the hard work, the social isolation and at last, the unhappy rupture and escape. His first marriage broke up, but in time he re-married and for the first time in our interviews, he admitted to hope and even a prospect of happiness.

Then his young daughter developed a malignancy, rare and aggressive and beyond all but fleeting relief. The experts did their best with heroic and horrendous therapy until she rebelled. It passed to me to make her deathly sick, rob her of hair and dignity and ease. It was my step that made her scream when I went to put the cannula into that wasted body.

She died in the local hospital in the presence of her family and family doctor.

Not many months later her mother too succumbed. She declined treatment. Who could blame her after what she had seen of it?

After many alarms, each of which posed for me the dilemma of resuscitation or release, she died at home.

The surviving children and their father somehow coped, although not without many social and domestic upheavals.

A little later on, my patient sustained an injury that left him physically impaired and, worse, robbed him of his only solace, searching in the wild for the gold so conspicuously missing from his life.

He would drift in to see me from time to time, always

unexpected and always accommodated. He took to worrying about his heart and, more for peace of mind for both of us than anything else, he was investigated, with negative results.

On the very night following his gastroscopy (we were still pursuing his chest pain) he called me for yet another one. With a diagnosis of oesophagitis made that afternoon, I opted for analgesia and reassurance and went back to bed. Two hours later I was back again. The ambulance joined us shortly afterwards.

Yes, it was in fact a big one they said and as soon as he was fit for it he was booked for by-pass surgery. It didn't go smoothly, of course. He developed a malignant arrhythmia with episodes of ventricular fibrillation terminating in asystole. In the end they got him to the super specialists and after much agonising on his part and encouragement from everyone else he had a mini-defibrillator implanted adjacent to the rebellious ventricle.

'Am I going to die?' he asked on his return and the answer was 'Yes, but only for a little while, then this thing in your chest will bring you to life again'. And with that reassurance he was urged to go back to 'normal' life again. For a while he haunted the local casualty departments and became a frequent flier with the ambulance service until he pinned his faith in a local consultant and (save the mark) me.

We had many anxious colloquies about his pulse rate and his blood pressure. I saw him without question as immediately as I could manage and when he came to me he waited on his own, for by now he shunned the company of others.

We discussed his terrors many times and he went via the physician to a psychologist who, by virtue of her own medical history, was uniquely suitable to understand him. We fiddled with anxiolytics and antidepressants, but what passes through a person's mind between asystole and reversion that a drug can block, or a counsellor can soothe away?

And now, if there were signs, I had missed them and he was dead. Somewhere, sometime, anxiety changed to despair and fear to resolution.

I think of the many times medicine touched that man's life: professorial units renal and cardiac, electrophysiologists and orthopaedic surgeons, rehabilitation teams, oncologists, physicians and psychologists. How many different pieces of his mind and body had engaged the attention of how many different doctors? I can scarcely claim membership of that distinguished team. At best, I was a sort of twelfth man, the one who occasionally fields in the deep, spends most of the time in the pavilion and carries the bag to the station. But he was on my special list.

And I was in at the death.

———————give me my staff

give me my staff ————————————————————

none other than ——————————————————————

but i don't want a nice day ————————————————

letters pray ——————————————————————

give me my staff

By the time I got back to the consulting room, she was down from the couch, dressed and seated. We discussed the problem (nothing very world shattering) and she rose to leave. As she passed the couch she paused, twitched the disordered sheet expertly smooth, squared the pillow and made for the door.

'Are you a nurse?' I asked.

'I was, 20 years ago. How did you know?'

They never lose it do they? The all-encompassing eye, the passion for neatness and exactitude, the ingrained distaste for inactivity, the inability to sit when there are things to be done, the reluctance to sit at all except for the snatched cup of coffee mid-session. Even then they look around for things to straighten and tidy up—their employers, for instance.

We always chose a nurse as our receptionist. Someone who could hold the fort when the partners were at lunch, calm the distracted, resist the demanding, placate the unreasonably angry and bring order to the daily chaos. They were good with the patients, too.

From time to time there were temporary non-nursing replacements. But so many of them, however brisk with the typewriter, however crisp on the telephone, blenched at the sight of blood and recoiled in horror from the messier accompaniments of general medical practice. They gave us our coffee on trays with little paper doilies, but treated every request for a visit as a major catastrophe and extracted us grumbling from a crowded surgery to clinical trivialities. And they expected someone else to mop up. If they stayed long enough they moved from awe-struck ignorance to breathtaking assurance and we heard with half an ear horrifying, one-sided conversations dispensing ill-adjudged advice, usually too late to intercept.

Then at last, at long last it seemed, she who must be admired returned to resume her sway and there was laughter again and order and very tidy couches.

Then surgery moved from the gloomy concrete arcade where

the toilet was known as 'the ice box', the dark room was under the stairs and stray rissoles from the cafe next door surfaced periodically in the wash tank, to custom-built splendour.

The staff had their own room, their own loo and their own mirror, selected by them and paid for, with little more than a stifled groan, by us. There were more and thicker carpets to be swept under her eye, more and shinier vinyl chairs to be polished when things were slack. We designed a desk, a masterpiece of ergonomic efficiency, high enough on the patient's side to stand and sign, low enough on the staff side to sit in comfort, within elbow reach of the telephone and arm's reach of the intercom. We even provided a chair specifically designed to cradle her back and wrap her shoulder blades in softly padded comfort.

She never sat in it. Every day I saw her leaning uncomfortably across the waist-high desk, crouching to murmur into the intercom, twisting painfully to reach the switchboard, all designed for access at a lower level. The bookkeeper annexed the chair. So, on slack afternoons she would perch uneasily on a battered kitchen stool that had somehow survived the modernisation. From time to time she would swoop on the empty waiting room to straighten the magazines, run a cloth over the chair seats or make a brisk pass with the carpet sweeper over the temporarily unoccupied floor.

But times changed. Our receptionist, our lynchpin, retired.

She helped us pick not one but two successors. It seemed politic to train two for the job that she had made her own. They, after all, were merely mortal.

We picked office workers. Sister concerned herself as always with clinical matters, but the front line, the shopfront, was no longer in the hands of a nurse. They slid smoothly into the unoccupied chairs, pivoting between telephone and screen. Files filled the shelves, filing trays were piled into high-rise plastic monuments of office efficiency and a baby hat stand sprouted rubber stamps. The typewriter clacked and chattered, the computer clicked and hummed and desk space was at a premium.

There were persuasive suggestions for more desks and more cleaners for the rather neglected carpets and slightly dishevelled couches. The whole place took on an air of purposeful sedentary activity.

I was reminded of all those articles about practice management, all those cash flow projections and budget forecasts, management reports and staff development programs. I recalled those afternoon sessions at so many seminars, when the clinical lecturers nicked off to the beach or the bazaar and left the rest of us to the blandishments of the accountants, financiers and marketing men. We heard ourselves described as small business managers, were gently denigrated as cottage industrialists and tactfully berated as peasants in the new exciting world of the entrepreneur.

The trouble was that I rather liked cottages. It might not be efficient to plod down the corridor to collect each patient from the waiting room, but it stretched the legs and cleared the head. Besides, you could pick up a surprising number of clinical clues watching them walk in front of you. It might not be dignified to stand the instrument cabinet on a po cupboard—fruit of a term's high school woodwork by my youngest—but it housed the telephone directories and spare handtowels and, of course, the po. It might not be politic to keep a quarter-inch masonry bit in the pen rack, but as a conversation piece it opened many a halting interview. There's no file like a largish blotter with urgent letters tucked under the front corner and invitations to practice management seminars hidden underneath.

Surely, inexorably, the new order will sweep these things away. Already, at one touch of a button I could telephone my partner in the room next door—so much less wear on the carpet, the door handle and the knuckles. Better still, at one touch of another button I could stop him or anybody else from telephoning me. Hooray for progress. Soon my po cupboard will be scrapped for something functional in stainless steel. Soon I shall forget that 'functional' means 'imaginary' in the clinical sense and hideously ugly in every other sense.

I have realised the essential difference between nurses who (like bar staff and traffic wardens) never sit and office workers who (like pianists and Olympic rowers) never stand.

But I don't complain. The staff wouldn't stand for it.

none other than

'And that is ...?' The voice was courteously interrogative if slightly ironical and I knew that another problem was on the way to solution.

The problems that face newly-hatched GPs are seldom clinical. They handle those with all the assurance of book learning unchastened by experience. It is the administrative blocks and personal quirks that madden. Between the cold logic of the system and the crazy unreason of the individual they struggle for an answer.

One of the horrors of my early years in practice was trying to get people into hospital. The practice straddled a county boundary and was on the fringe of three hospital catchment areas, which multiplied the prospect of denial by three and the number of necessary telephone calls by six.

I crouched shivering in a telephone box, laden with small change and spoke to a succession of haughty residents, while an inevitable abortion down the street soaked steadily through the bedclothes and relays of anxious relatives rattled on the window. It was the GP's common lot in those benighted days, and I remember one of my colleagues making the headlines by smashing a public telephone in sheer frustration and being hauled, still blaspheming, before the magistrate.

Then I discovered Mr Greenslade and my problems were solved. He, God bless him, was the night switch at our nearest and least co-operative hospital and it was to him I confided my problems. Thanks to his suave and efficient manipulation my patients were thereafter admitted without question or delay.

After a while he got to know my voice and would preface his suggestions with 'And that is none other than ...?'.

He was one of that select band of intermediaries—the senior NCOs, the chief porters, the supervisors, the clerk of works—the vital noiseless cogs, the invisible wheels that make any organisation work.

Nowadays, no doubt, they would be called 'middle management', but their management reaches to every squeaking spindle in the corporate machine.

It was he who knew where the empty beds were and where the resident had taken refuge. He even threw in little character sketches to help with my pleas. 'She's a lady, Sir ', he'd say or 'He's Irish, but quite helpful' and indicate the most fruitful line of approach—imperious or fawning, jocular or anxious, as the case required. He was courteous but never servile, helpful but never officious. I wonder if he knew just what I owed him in personal balance and domestic harmony.

I hadn't thought of him for years until quite recently, when a telephone call reminded me that he and his kind are still, thank God, at work. The telephone call was from the secretary of one of our local visiting gurus who, on his monthly visit, had seen and agreed to excise a nasty little lesion from a special patient. Special because she had watched her husband die of just such a lesion, which ran wild and finally ate its way from his cheek to the base of his brain despite the best efforts of the experts. I was anxious for her to jump the waiting list and short-circuit the inevitably cumbrous processes of the public hospital system, battling as it must the many demands for priority.

'I've read your letter', she said.

'Mr Blank is away but we must get your patient in as soon as he gets back. I'll talk to the girls in admission and put her on his first list. Only don't tell her until it's official.'

And now she's home again, that special patient, relieved of her lesion and, one hopes, her dread. And her doctor reaps undeserved bouquets that belong to the surgeon and still more to his secretary and to that underground network of compassion and common sense that adapts the system to the user.

Underlying all the necessary structure of health care, unrecognised by any fee schedule, unacknowledged by any statutory award, there is an elite who make it work. It is not sufficient for them to know the procedures, follow the protocols or observe the regulations—any collection of printed circuits and microchips can do that. What is important is for them to adapt, interpret, improvise and understand the human problems that they are here to cater for.

Hospitals are built for the sick not the staff; surgeries are geared for service not income. When it is the other way around, not only does the care suffer, but the carers too become disenchanted and disgruntled.

Even in this cynical and greedy age, some people find fulfilment in giving more than a wage is worth, a clock measures or a tariff values. By an odd paradox, those who give more gain more and take their profits in gratitude, esteem and inward satisfaction.

I'm not advocating a return to some sort of monastic dedication to poverty and abnegation, a total surrender to the sick and querulous, although I guess that's how it may have started.

A complacent reliance on amiability and good intention can stultify progress, conceal ignorance and protect ineptitude. It is science that salvages tiny babies, care that makes it worthwhile. 'Wage justice', that cant phrase, does mean something more than greed and working to rule.

Let us be just to ourselves, as long as we are also just to our patients and faithful to our principles. But whether we swing to some mystical muddle of compassion or turn to the stern realities of technology, whether our hospitals turn into churches or factories, offices or laboratories, we still need and still have Mr Greenslade and his ilk.

We can still reach someone in the lower branches of the ever-growing administrative tree who can help.

I don't know what they paid him, my invaluable friend—not enough, I'm sure. Nor, I suspect, are the services of that understanding medical secretary justly compensated. But if either of them should happen on this tribute I hope they will accept it in part recognition of their worth.

It comes from the heart of 'None other than …'.

but i don't want a nice day

There are quite strict rules about telephone calls in our practice—who leaves or receives messages; who telephones or is telephoned back; who is put through without question. In this latter privileged group are colleagues in the widest sense, a category that includes, or should I say embraces: nurses, pharmacists, preachers, undertakers, gently reproachful editors, patients on the social circuit and those brazen telephonic bulldozers who breeze down the wire at inopportune moments with offers of instant wealth.

I think it was the last group who originated the technique of offering only a first name (not 'given', they get that from me later). It takes someone tougher than our receptionist to obstruct Kevin from Collins Street or Maribell of Martin Place. So, within seconds of the imperious buzz, I have dropped the speculum, daubed the handset with Hibitane cream and found myself rejecting with increasing irritation ten thousand dollars of illusory capital gain. Caught, as it were, with someone else's trousers down and anxiously trying to preserve that suavity that marks the true professional, it is all too easy to give the soft answer. It takes at least a month afterwards to convince Maribell that buying escudos on a falling market to acquire heating oil on a rising market to sell to Eskimos on a freezing market, is not my recipe for early retirement.

My particular persecutor finally dropped his hollow joviality and snapped, 'Aren't you interested in making money?' How satisfying the reply: 'I'm trying to, if only you'd get off the bloody line.' Game, set and match to me—a rare victory.

The contagion of meaningless intimacy is spreading. I'm delighted to learn that the local insurance office telephonist is Linda and she cheerily asks, can she help me? Yes she can, by putting me through to her boss. But does she? Oh no. He is on his second Friday or paternity leave or his knees or the other line. Would I like to talk to Fred (accounts), Doreen (typing pool), Ben (gardener). No? Then thank you for calling and have a nice day.

I don't want a nice day. I want someone who will permit me to explain my problem without interrupting, comprehend it and answer it alone or after consulting the appropriate expert. I am not calling to brighten Linda's day or pass a casual hour listening to a glutinous glockenspiel while the boss is on another line. A day spent this way can scarcely be called nice.

Telephoning a hospital, of course, is different. No nice days there, just a distant hauteur, like a butler of the old school and a swift merciless telephonic triage to surgical west or medical three. 'Mr Brown is on his round and I'll put you back to switch.' Round one and there are many more to go. It has all the verve of Monopoly, this game of 'put you back to switch', except that you never pass 'Go', still less collect two hundred dollars. You slither down the telephone totem from consultant (in a meeting), to registrar (on study leave), to resident (in theatre), holding the line betweenwhiles like a drowning man, ever shuttling back to switch until you pour your story into a sympathetic ear, which turns out to belong to the kiosk lady in outpatients.

I will admit that our staff are not guiltless in this regard. 'What was the name again?' they ask, as if Jones has turned to Robinson while the caller waited. And 'Which Mrs Brown?'. That must be a poser at the other end. Does she say 'The one with two heads' or 'That woman whose wretched kids pooped in the passageway last week'? I never like to ask.

But I don't think they play the super secretary game. The one that goes 'I bet I can get your boss to the telephone before mine'. You know the sequence—the crisp introduction, 'Dr A, it's Dr B calling', then the fatal phrase 'Hold on'. To what? The telephone, your hat, your sanity? Then a volley of clicks, a barrage of buzzes and silence. The pause that follows is presumably for you to remove the other rubber glove, straighten your tie and adjust your thoughts for the awesome message to come. 'Connecting you now', wait for it, more clicks, more chirps and buzzes, a querulous 'Yes' from the other end and you open the conversation with a wholly unnecessary apology.

Doctors' telephone answering techniques are a study in themselves. New residents cower behind their boss's eminence, older ones announce themselves with curt clarity, GPs offer soft 'Hellos', brisk in youth, wary in middle age and resigned in later years. Consultants pay someone else to do it for them.

The relentless march of technology that replaced the exchange girls' personal tinkle with the soulless double clangour of a machine has moved on now to distant and discreet cosmic pippings or barely audible warbles as an excuse to interrupt your work and invade your leisure. You can dial a recipe, or a Test score and, in the event of disaster in either case, a prayer: it will be a remedy next, no doubt.

You can hide your telephone in a radio, flaunt it in your car, slip it into your pocket, take it on picnics or leave it at home to lie for you, but it shatters your sleep at 3.00 a.m. just the same.

After a night or two of that, who looks forward to a nice day?

letters pray

Nowadays, of course, nobody talks or writes—they *communicate*. They talk *with* never to others and hold meaningful dialogue at all levels. The latter phrase conjures up a pleasing picture of simultaneous monologues, delivered now on the floor, now on the table, now at the top of a 12-foot ladder. Argument has become a matter of confrontation, eyeball to eyeball, although I would have thought kneecap to kneecap offered greater scope for emphatic gesture. But we still have to write letters to one another from time to time and then the fun really starts.

The discerning student of intermedical communication (iatrograffics should I call it?) recognises many classes of correspondence. There are the PS&Ts—please see and treats. These are handwritten, occasionally on headed notepaper, more often on high quality wrapping paper and the only easily legible information is the date (which you know already) and perhaps the name of the patient (which you can usually find out for yourself). At the bottom a mark rather than a signature is all too familiar to the hapless casualty officer who is the usual target.

There are variations that include anatomical details (my favourite was 'Query legs', to which the only possible rejoinder is 'Legs present') or pathological speculation, such as '?Appendicitis' and the answer, 'What, again?'

Sometimes it seems to the harassed resident that some practices run only on Valium and visiting cards. The outpatients at my teaching hospital was largely supported by two amiable souls from the neighbouring lock-up surgery, who relied on an annual Christmas party to mollify a year's frustration. I remember the day when a testy ENT consultant dictated his end-of-session letter, 'Dear Drs X & Y, thank you for your morning surgery'.

The hospital riposte to this sort of letter is a pro-forma. This tells you, two weeks after the event, that your patient has been discharged today (ha, ha), having recovered normally from an appendicectomy and is on no medication (which is a pity, because he is a diabetic who has been on the verge of cardiac failure for the last five years) and that a more detailed letter will follow.

Next comes the terse one line referral, usually surgical, which actually says 'For God's sake, take this child's tonsils out before she drives me mad' and the equally terse reply 'My registrar will, when we are good and ready'.

Letters to physicians take longer and indeed, like X-ray or histology reports, their length is inversely proportional to the certainty. 'I'm pretty sure' takes half a page or so, 'I think' spreads on to a second sheet and 'I'm hopelessly at sea' involves three or four foolscap sheets. Replies from these august personages may be classified as:

(a) the suavely upstage: 'You fool, if you'd taken a decent history and actually examined someone for a change you would see that the answer is staring you in the face';
(b) the blandly non-committal: 'I've ordered half a dozen obscure investigations which you won't know about and with any luck the patient will have got better or produced some decent physical signs by the time they come back';
(c) the maddeningly tangential: 'Thank you for referring Mrs Blank with varicose veins. I noted an elevated blood pressure and have ordered a vast battery of tests and sent her on to my colleague Dr Y'.

There is a special tone to the enforced referral letter. The one that says, 'I know perfectly well what's wrong with this stupid man and am quite capable of treating it, but he insists on a specialist and of all people he's picked you'. And no doubt our specialist colleagues recognise the GP cry for help, 'I know there's nothing wrong with her and so will you, but please convince her and don't despise me for wasting your time'.

Now we all have dictating machines and secretaries, and if we have the College system, rational notes. The temptation to prolixity and irrelevance is strong. Longhand is terse but illegible and even dictation has pitfalls. I will never know whether the typist who transmuted 'below knee' into 'boloney' was inattentive or scornful.

The ultimate in progress is the print out—a massive screed covered with the alien typography of the computer, which is unstoreable in conventional offices. Computers can be polite if not witty, but they never seem to know when to stop.

Correspondence to and from psychiatrists is in a field of its own. Most of us feel obliged to spread ourselves when writing to someone whose business is words and few can resist slipping the occasional pejorative adjective that reveals more of the writer than the subject. The reply is long, informative, elegantly phrased and defies abridgement. They unearth details that have remained hidden in a decade of personal care and contact, they occasionally suggest, or what is worse uncover, organic illness and all appear to work on the principle that medication without striking side effects is pointless.

The first dystonic reaction to phenothiazine I met sent me flying to the telephone, pursued by an incoherent patient apparently trying to undo his tie with his tongue. The specialist, when eventually contacted, was interested but slightly blasé and the suggested antidote was gratifyingly effective. Powerful medicine which dispelled my patient's baseless anxieties—and added to mine.

Sometimes, you send your patient duly documented, appropriately investigated, to an expert and both vanish. From time to time, the patient reappears, seeking off-work certificates or fresh referral notes, or summons you in the small hours to cope with the side effects of a drug you've never used, prescribed by a consultant you've never heard of. Cryptic messages reach you periodically from unexpected sources until the patient drifts out of your ken.

But the most aggravating of all is the letter that never comes, or arrives after the funeral. I have a patient whose renal failure I followed for nearly seven years. We plodded together down the disheartening trail of disability, the progressive decisions of whether, then when and finally how, to dialyse. We enlisted the local paper and the local Lions Club and sundry state authorities and got a machine for him and a caravan to put it in.

His wife, who fainted at the sight of blood, found herself needling his arteries three times a week, while his doctor looked on and shuddered. Heparinised blood makes fascinating patterns on a caravan wall.

His doctor added two pints of blood to the circuit when the haemoglobin sank to 5G and put it on the wrong side. Have you ever seen a drip running upwards? I have. Intercurrent infect ions were a nightmare and there were one or two hasty trips to the renal unit 200 miles away.

They started talking transplants and his name was added to the list. The long-awaited summons was dramatic when at last it came—a telegram in the early hours, a hurried plane trip the following day.

Then one day he appeared at the surgery, puffy with prednisolone, radiant with cheerfulness, on his way back to the referring renal unit.

And how did his doctor know about his operation, his medication, his future management and his likely progress? It was in the local paper.

Perhaps I should have written to them for the clinical notes.

———————off and away

time off

'you was away'

why fishing?

anti-social climbing

overseas and overspent

small change

more than a month of sundays

time off

It had to happen. Now that there were four of us it was simple arithmetic that each of us would have one night call per week and one weekend off in a month. Before then, it had been two night calls per week and even before that, we were all on-call all of the time, except for our precious half-day. It was a matter of some pride in those early days that you cared for your own most of the time. Each of us felt, no doubt with some pride, that he and he alone was in demand. We bore our burden of dedication with a secret pride that did nothing to mute the midnight telephone.

It was part of the ethos, the mystique of medicine, that doctors didn't keep office hours and didn't watch the clock.

As a resident there was an almost military feeling—a sense of comradeship in an endless campaign; a total involvement in the rigours and demand of the hospital world.

You compared your lot with lesser breeds who had their evenings free, whose every weekend belonged to them alone, who slammed the office door on their day's work in the late afternoon, who took time off to go to the races, or could catch the flu without shame or penalty. You scorned those who must be bribed with extra pay to complete a job, just as you scoffed aloud at the notion of dedication.

But secretly, you preened yourself, revelled in the notion of your indispensability and your importance in the scheme of things. On those sporadic forays into the outside world for a non-medical party or a long overdue haircut, you looked with kindly contempt on those who talked of things other than medicine, who did not know, worse still did not wish to know, the password to your private cosmos.

Then, at last, the just claims of junior doctors were recognised and rewarded. Overtime *was* paid, night duty became night shift and there was time to join that outside world.

It was the same in practice. The advent of a newcomer to a two-handed practice allowed the principals to spend time with their families, work in the garden or go to the opera. How well I remember my principal saying this to me. Up to that point he had had one evening free a week with alternate Saturdays and Sundays off and before then, no relief at all. 'And do you know', he said, 'the moment I handed my practice over to somebody else, even for half a day, I lost something'. I nodded sympathetically and privately thought he was nuts. But not as nuts as the other partner who felt guilty about no longer holding a surgery on Sundays.

Now in my turn I feel not exactly guilty, but just a little wistful and certainly not dismayed about the changes in my professional life.

What have I gained? Three, more often than not six, certain nights of uninterrupted sleep per week and a corresponding expansion in leisure time and social freedom. Time to devote to the family, cut the grass, wash the car and fix the washing machine.

What have I lost? The ability to grab the telephone at the first ting, awake, alert and orientated; the determination to use every available second of my precious time off productively; the handy alibi for dull dinner parties.

But my family has grown up and gone away, I loathe gardening and I would rather go to church than wash the car. If this is the ease and freedom I so envied in accountants and solicitors and other nine-to-fivers, I wonder what all the fuss was about.

True, I now have the chance to attend weekend seminars on total patient care, addressed by experts who do even less out-of-hours work than I do. But, by the strange perversity of human nature, where I once could and did spare precious sparse off-duty time for such worthy objects, now from the comparative freedom of a much lighter schedule I resent any professional intrusion.

I have discovered too some of the drawbacks of shared care. It is much more difficult to resist a continuing nightly demand for opiates when it is only your problem once a week. The chance of defusing or exploring a family crisis varies inversely with your involvement. The prospect of bowing out at eight o'clock next morning, alluring as it is, can postpone or compound a problem that sooner or later will have to be confronted by somebody. You can't get by with casual medicine for casualties.

Mind you, I'm as devious as the next in dodging if I can get away with it. On those occasions when conscience and a little connubial pressure drives me to respond to pleas that I could legitimately divert, I leave home in a sulphurous cloud, however unctuous I may be on arrival at the stricken house—and there is a little virtuous glow—until the next time. In short, I want to be needed, not not to be called. So, I suspect, do most of my colleagues.

We like to think that our interest lingers after the clock has struck, we like to believe that we still sacrifice time and sleep when it is asked of us, we like to feel a little bit more involved than the rest.

Is that the time? I should have been off-duty half an hour ago.

'you was away'

She heaved a sigh that stirred the tiers of her chins.

'I came last week', she said reproachfully, 'but you was away'.

'You could have seen my locum, he was very good' (I think).

'Oh him.'

We've only had locums for the past few years, only in fact since we stopped playing 'I can go longer without a break than you can' in the practice. I must say it is nice not to pay for your vacation by working twice as hard when you get back.

Your partner's patients are such strange people and his therapy so bizarre. If you see them in his absence you feel exploited, if they prefer to wait for his return you feel slighted. But a hired hand has his or her drawbacks. First, there is all the business of finding one. We don't live in a city ceaselessly patrolled by unemployed registrars in radio-controlled limousines complete with cardiograph and cash register. Nor are we adjacent to a bleep of residents prepared to slum it occasionally so they can buy their second campervan.

We put the word around, rejecting as kindly as possible the

nonagenarian colleagues who retired 20 years ago and not before time. We pursued the summer transients last heard of in Bangladesh. We answer advertisements from 'muscular Christians' ('no surgery, midwifery, or anaesthetics'), 'globetrotting Edinburgh academics' ('have linear accelerator will travel') or 'fully-experienced GPs' who graduated six months ago (no way surgery, midwifery, anaesthetics or anything else in my practice).

Eventually, the bread upon the waters returns. First, a telephone call on a bad line, beat music their end, howling babies yours. Later, a more coherent conversation when dates and rates are chaffered. Accommodation? Certainly. A car? Naturally. Time off? Within reason. Weekends? Just the one. Fares for self, wife, baby and goat from Alice Springs? Reluctantly.

If he or she is local there are rumours. Isn't that the one who wears earrings/organised a work-to-rule/keeps bees/ran away with the dietician?

The local consultants admit to hazy remembrance. 'Yes, I think they worked for me—to some extent. Try to get them to wash occasionally.' Or through pursed lips, 'I remember them very well. [Pause] Will you be away long?'

There is an interview: slightly hollow-heartiness on our side, slightly bogus confidence on his or hers.

The staff react. They think he/she's 'gorgeous' or 'all right, I suppose'. They comment, 'After all, jeans do suit the younger man' or 'All that make-up and did you see her shoes?'.

Evening comes. The car is loaded, then unloaded to fetch the locum (and family). The dog is introduced and reprimanded for discourtesy, the house and fittings are revealed, the vagaries of the plumbing disclosed and the state of the second car frankly admitted. Your wife urges them, rather unnecessarily you feel, to make themselves at home. The car is reloaded.

Next morning, there is a flurry of introductions, a slightly defensive résumé of outstanding clinical and social problems and a hurried tour of the facilities. Then, amidst grateful adieux and final directions about cat food and hairdressers, you drive away.

The feeling of guilt at leaving your patients and partners in such unknown hands evaporates at the town boundary; concern for the cat and dog you left behind lasts a little longer.

Locums come in so many different sizes and types. Young or old, trendy or drab, diffident or confident. Some pass through leaving no visible mark but unidentifiable handwriting and a penchant for costly medication. Some leave enduring monuments of gratitude or disaster, an anthology of anecdotes, a catalogue of mannerisms. Some ask advice—flattering when you're slack, irritating when you're busy, maddening when you have none to give. Some slip quietly in and out without disturbance or remark. Some stall, defer decisions and refer for needless opinions from unrespected sources.

Others ruthlessly disorganise the illness you have patiently organised over many years. Some leave behind a mound of asymptomatic and untreatable biochemical abnormalities and a heap of negative findings that have stretched your local laboratory to the limit. Some openly admire your practice, some gently criticise and some are wisely silent.

We have had MRACPs fresh from ICU and retired consultants weary from the labour ward. We have had those who vanished at the stroke of five and those who spent half the night discussing clinical problems of (to them) absorbing interest. We have had those who reacted to all crises by summoning an ambulance and those whose heroic manoeuvres puzzled and alarmed our local hospital. They have all added something and perhaps taken something away, have taught something and perhaps learnt something.

Two weeks later you re-enter your house. It is ablaze with light, loud with unexpected music and pungent with exotic cooking smells. The dog growls, the cat—suspiciously sleek—sidles away from your stroking hand. Your guest is on the telephone.

To New York? No, to the hospital, issuing crisp instructions for equipment you have never heard of and drugs you dare not use. There have been no problems ... except — and you are pleased to find that some of your clinical enigmas are enigmas still.

As the tan fades and the pace quickens, you develop a grudging respect for this unknown who has shed new light on your problems, has left behind—with the fused kettle and alien socks—new avenues, different perspectives and—dare you admit it—better solutions. An untried stranger has invaded your domain and left behind a trail of new drugs and the occasional startling but retrospectively obvious diagnosis, by following leads hitherto ignored and clues heretofore overlooked.

It's strange to hear your patients' comments on someone you know solely as a hole in the bank balance and a burn in the sitting room carpet.

It's stranger still when patients arrive demanding appointments with the *new* doctor, the *young* doctor, not with you.

You was away.

why fishing?

I wonder why it is that so many of my colleagues escape from the cares of clinical practice to the riverbank. What is it about the simple act of conning one of God's creatures into swallowing an illusory meal and an all-too-real hook and dragging it by the throat from its natural habitat to garnish a frying pan or grace a mantelshelf?

Strange behaviour indeed from a group of men and women who claim to care. That those who spend the other 50 weeks of the year trying to heal others, applying their hard-won talents for patient persuasion, deft manoeuvre and swift reaction, should take a positive pleasure in matching cunning for cunning and greed for greed in pursuit of the blameless citizens of a different world.

Or is it so strange? Every holiday is an escape, but no one flees without some luggage, if only the habit of their usual life. How often in the consulting room do we cast a bait before a reluctant confidant, invite a patient to share a secret dread or uncover innermost feelings?

We sit by the stream, watching for the telltale ripples and flicking a tempting fly to invite confidences and confidence. As with angling, there are more bites than successes and many a time the patient you are gently steering towards health or understanding will slip stealthily away. And you look over your tackle, ponder your technique and curse perhaps your quarry, perhaps the gods, but the creel is empty.

Or is it the latent sadism that years of professional suppression have not wholly vanquished that spices your triumphant captures?

Is it the personal, almost vindictive, pleasure of bending another to your will, of calling the tune for once? You pay for it with many empty hours and disappointed hopes, but for a few glorious moments you are omnipotent.

Those hours of waiting, far from the telephone, baggily garbed, uncomfortably perched, also bring their own rewards. You are free to wander lazily through your mind, picking and discarding stray thoughts not worth the effort of connection, basking in the sunlight (if there is any) and enduring the rain (as rain there mostly is), until the boat runs aground, the beer goes flat and the belly looks for something more substantial. And you potter back to camp, cook your meal, lie about your exploits and crawl contentedly to bed.

I suppose other professions take their pleasures in other ways. Do accountants visit their brothers of the turf? Do they put in doubtful returns over the net? Do engineers build sandcastles or play bridge? Do lawyers adjourn to casinos or execute deeds on water skis? Do social workers purge 11 months of endless patience and sympathetic understanding with a fortnight in the city mugging old people? Do teachers—but come, what else do they do?

For a week or two you slip into another world and another skin. You cast off the habitual shackles of your daily round and escape. For a little while you can be a jetsetter or a pioneer, you can play the tables or the field, lounge or leap, choose burial in the country or cremation in town, until your partners are exasperated and the credit card is exhausted.

For me, that other world is remote and redolent of wood smoke and brown trout—a place of huge unhealthy meals and strange unlikely hours. It has its customs, its privileges and even its secrets. Entry to that select company of the initiated is not readily offered or easily earned. It is, thank God, a million miles away from medicine, although I have learned to carry with me enough instruments to extract hooks and antacids to sooth whisky-washed oesophagi. I used to take a whole dispensary of needless drugs, but nowadays time and senescence have equipped most of my companions with enough cardiac and respiratory medicaments to start a clinic on the riverbank.

There is less enthusiasm for dawn starts these days and a growing reluctance to battle the elements. Given enough dry wood, a cribbage board and a can or two, some of the best fish are caught by the fire, again—and again.

So, as you make for the Gold Coast or head for Bangkok, pack the gear for the snow or the shorts for the beach, think of me. Better still, as you trudge to the clinic or crawl out of bed, spare a thought for the trout that is coming aboard.

At a rough estimate, it will have cost 30 or 40 dollars a pound (we still measure in them down our way). It will have been long awaited, judiciously played, cunningly netted and royally welcomed. A precious beast indeed. If its remaining career is short, hot and savoury, its memory will see me through a dozen disappointments in the months to come and its kindred will call me back a dozen months from now.

If you're looking for me at the end of the month, I'll be away fishing among all the pleasures of the bush and the comforts of the camp. I'll be 40 miles from a telephone and a thousand miles from the job. There will be no journals, rounds or regrets and—best of all—no deadlines.

They're illegal.

anti-social climbing

I wouldn't describe myself as an active exerciser, still less a mountaineer. This walk was a mere seven hours in duration and nine miles in length, with a two thousand feet rise and, more to the point, fall, but for a man who restricts his jogging to memory, his walking to twice weekly ambles around the block after the dog and his running to occasional bath water, it was something of a challenge.

But, after all, I was (for the time being) a non-smoker. The whole thing should have been a breeze.

It was. A breeze that rasped painfully between clenched teeth, while the sweat trickled merrily between the shoulder blades and distant muscles painfully complained. True, I no longer tasted the tarry residues of last night's pipe, but the piquant flavour of this morning's smoked oysters was equally unpalatable. Strange nutriment you will say for mountain climbing, but I am not really experienced in these matters.

Professional cyclists and other Olympian masochists talk of the 'pain barrier'. Actually, it's the coaches and commentators who talk of it, the performers merely suffer and breach it in agonising silence. I think I reached it, but not before passing through the 'puff barrier', the 'purge barrier', the 'puke barrier' and other alliterative and unmentionable cries of alarm from an outraged carcase. For the first time in 30-odd years, I re-lived the sensations of a sluggish rugby forward in the 13th minute of a seven-a-side game, when the spring sun is high, the scores are level and extra time is inevitable.

It was, in retrospect, a mistake to have read and remembered the editorial (*MJA*) on sudden death and exercise, but as the track steepened and the knees weakened my mood changed from grim foreboding to almost eager anticipation. That line about 'full half in love with easeful death' ran pleasantly through my head.

I made it (the summit, that is), spurred on by pride, hitherto unexpanded alveoli and long overlooked hoards of glycogen. My companions sauntered airily ahead and I lurched uncertainly from rock to rock, lured on by successive summits that melted away as each fresh pitch came into view.

At the very top we rested. The sky proved to be blue, not black with intermittently twinkling stars as it had seemed on the way up, and the views were magnificent.

I discovered that water is a very good drink in its time and place and marvelled at the men who had built and cemented the cairn at the top. How, I wondered, had they carted the materials, as well as themselves, to such a place—trained with tins of smoked oysters, no doubt.

Then we descended, quartering the mountain slopes on tremulous legs and strained to reach the valley below before the sun left it first. It now seemed possible that I would last long enough to reach cold beer and hot water. The crepe bandage I sneaked into my kit bag could be sneaked back into the surgery unsullied; the helicopter could stay at home.

The last 50 steps (cruel postscript) were climbed foot by leaden foot. Then we reached the cars and the cans and life was good.

On the drive home it was interesting and anatomically testing to predict and identify which muscle groups would go into spasm next and to work out anatomically and physiologically the optimum resting position to defeat their malevolent intent. In fact, it was not easy—physi it may have been, logical it was not.

Trial and error provided the ultimate solution: right foot on the clutch, left foot through the passenger window, resting on the aerial. It proved impractical, especially as I was sitting in the passenger seat. My driver calmly remarked that cramp was largely overcome by willpower: if you detected the onslaught early enough you could prevent it by sheer force of character. It was, she said, mostly in the mind, though I was more inclined to place it in the hamstrings, no the adductors, or maybe the gastrocnemius or, by God, the glutei.

It passed and I remembered about heatstroke and salt tablets, quinine and Valium or, at a pinch (ha), gin and tonic.

In the end it was whisky internally, hot water externally and a happy haze of fatigue, repletion and slumber.

My middle-aged body subsided happily into its accustomed torpor, leaving occasional aching reminders in the legs and a week-long reluctance to rise from the desk.

Exercise? I can take it or leave it. I didn't drop dead. I don't think I was fit enough, but there are many more comfortable ways to achieve that and I might even try it again.

But I shall take it with a pinch of salt next time.

overseas and overspent

Conference going is a singular pastime. Some go as a guilty compromise between postgraduate education and family recreation, slipping away to lectures while the spouse drowses by the pool and the children squabble in it; a privileged few go to speak; an eager handful go to listen; and an awkward clique go to argue. Some seek enlightenment and some escape; all expect relief—of tax, or tension or other things.

Visiting gurus of the medical caste lose all dignity in shrunken shoes and shirts that would excite comment even in Hawaii. Distinguished surgeons are found to have impressive golf handicaps; erudite physicians display a fine taste in wines and a predilection for lurid paperbacks; world-class paediatricians loudly reprimand their own and other people's children; and dermatologists get frightful sunburn.

A sense of shame impels you from time to time to lectures in motel dining rooms, where the microphone doesn't work but the slide projector, alas, does. There, barricaded away from the tropical sunshine and excluded from the tropical trade winds you swelter the morning away, peeling burnt and sweaty skin from relentless plastic chairs, while happy cries from the swimming pool and a distant clink of misted glasses in the bar mock the whole futile exercise.

And at the finish, addresses are exchanged (and lost) and promises are lightly made (and broken). What little learning you have garnered slips away to join the huge catalogue of subjects you really must find out about—some other time.

The best conferences are overseas conferences. Foreign rooms are always cheaper in baht or rupiah and the continental breakfast they throw in (often quite literally) blinds you to the expense of eating for the rest of the time, to say nothing of other outgoings. Not even the miraculous bamboo of the tropics grows as quickly overnight as a burgeoning bar bill.

I once attended two overseas conference in less than 12 months. Neither was in the tropics. Flinders Island (the first) is about as far South of the tropic of Capricorn as London (the second) is North of the tropic of Cancer and I expect there are other significant differences.

I didn't know how strong the CWA was in London, but I bet Flinders had them beat pavlova-wise. A Guildhall banquet is all very well, but give me Flinders Golf Club any day. Where else in the world could I have shared my bread roll with the snotty offspring of a garrulous if half-witted ex-patient, who dropped in for a chat between the soup and the stroganoff? A free pass on the London Underground didn't have quite the same distinction as half a seat on a minibus directed by the local Minister of Health. It gave new meaning to the term steering committee.

Certainly I found London a little more cosmopolitan. There were speakers there from Finland, Haiti, Panama and Israel, for instance—but there was a chap on Flinders who *said* he came from Sydney. And you would expect a wider coverage in London from the, and I quote, World Organisation of National Colleges, Academies and Academic Associations of General Practitioners/Family Physicians (very important that '/'). At the Guildhall affair the coffee was stone-cold before the after-dinner speaker had even named the organisation, let alone toasted it.

This comprehensive title covers a vast assemblage ranging, I discovered, from the polyclinicians of New York City to the beleaguered generalists of Bangladesh. I must have fitted in there somewhere, perhaps in the '/' between GPs and Family Physicians.

If the title is difficult to rattle off without pausing for breath, the acronym is scarcely fit for polite company. When I first confessed to Marylou, the travel agent so thoughtfully recommended by the College (offering six per cent discount on the normal fares), that I planned to attend a conference of WONCA's in London, she was inclined to recommend Sweden as a likelier venue for that sort of thing.

The first one I attended, in about 1974 I think, was in Melbourne. There was no Marylou, or minibus, but I have vague recollections of caged snakes in the foyer, complimentary South Australian wines in the corridor and a visiting Yankee in the auditorium who said 'problemorientedmedicalrecords' as one word. I wonder what happened to him, or his records? The theme then was 'Medicine in the Year 2000' and it seemed, I remember, to involve computers (not in my time, I said), physicians' aides, which in those days meant people not viruses (not in my practice, I said) and leading teams of paramedicals—or was it allied health personnel? (not in my town, I said). I went away burdened with brochures, saturated with South Australian wine and all for WONCA.

Since then, that organisation has WONCA'd all over the place, from New Orleans to Alma-Ata and many a town besides. This year it settles for a week in London and addresses itself to 'Towards 2000'. Getting closer you see. I don't know what fresh enthusiasms and startling insights I shall bring back in my luggage, but it won't be mutton birds. You only get them on Flinders.

small change

It was the longest, busiest and by far the most expensive holiday of my life. I left the clinical cares to others and vanished. I left the pens, the visiting diary, the surgery keys (but not, of course, the credit cards or wallet) behind, doffed the blazer, dropped the newspapers and turned a T-shirted back on the continuity of care and the inner consultation. I became not a tourist of course, but a traveller.

Timetable in one hand, phrasebook in the other ('Constable my wife has lost her goblets—no windows—ah, I see, glasses'. What, I wonder, is the Spanish for 'Up yours too, mate'?), camera unobtrusively slung, I became an atom, or rather a molecule, for my wife was always there to pack and repack the ever-more bulging grips and translate alien prices into cold Aussie dollar reality. Together we joined the busy bloodstream of Western Europe.

I wish I could say that I visited distinguished colleagues, hurried through health centres and sat at the feet of the eminent. And in a sense I did. But the colleagues I visited were mostly grey-haired and retired and more concerned with growing roses; the health centres I marvelled at were the lavish accidents of government largesse—all glowing terminals and parquetry flooring; and the only eminence my otherwise undistinguished year produced was dead.

I got so far away from medicine that to go any further would have been to come back. Even so, you cannot entirely shut away reflections on your livelihood. Perhaps it was the repeated experience of pacing busy streets unrecognised and unregarded, of being accountable to no one for my whereabouts, of knowing only the impersonal solicitude of those who wanted my money and their abrupt disinterest when they'd got it, that turned my thoughts sometimes to home.

I began to miss the kindly interest of the neighbours in my little town. I won't say I pined, but sometimes while queuing in some foreign eating house I thought wistfully of our accustomed table at the steak house and the welcome that goes with it, for which no charge is levied and no VAT is demanded. I missed the cheery 'good mornings' in the street, mostly from bad debts, the long quasi-clinical gossips with partners, the mandatory digest from the barber and the sense of consequence. Yes, that was what I missed—status.

I started to ask myself, in the small hours after the paella and the ill-advised Black Forest Cake, 'Who the hell are you anyway?'. An ageing bourgeois with thinning hair and thickening waist, a small-town, small-time professional, not learned enough to be a lawyer, or smart enough to be an accountant.

'My dear fellow', I answered, as I made for the toilet, again, 'I am a GP'.

'So what?'

So what, indeed. Often swinging sleeplessly through the night on some continental train, peering beneath the blind at yet another foreign station called 'Hommes', I tried to answer that question. It's such an odd job we do. We cultivate our little patch, sorting through the trivialities of medicine, panning the sands of the commonplace for the tiny specks of clinical gold that make the day worthwhile. Always looking for that rare unarguable triumph or the patient resolution of a multi-stranded knot, for genuine gratitude genuinely deserved, merit respected and for once, rewarded.

We deal so much in the small change of medicine that our learned colleagues may forget that over a lifetime it adds up to a goodly sum. It becomes such a habit to see our work as coughs and colds and the comfort of those who will not fit into clinical categories, that in the end we believe it ourselves.

But who, I asked myself, will miss me in the surgery? Will any of my patients be one penny the worse off for the absence of their family doctor? Only my locum perhaps, battling through illegibility to the inexplicable, gleefully unearthing my omissions and misapprehensions, bringing some order to my muddled therapeutics. And he may feel, though he is far too polite to say, none are worse and some are a darned sight better.

My local consultants will be just as grateful for his 'very helpful letter' as they claim to be for mine; his signature on a sickie carries no less weight; his tactful pleas for telephones or council housing will be just as politely disregarded. His morning tea will be no less fragrant—probably more so, in fact, as he supplies his own Lapsang Souchong (I don't mind that, but he takes it away with him afterwards)—and the fickle staff fawn and flatter him, never me. Or so I believe.

He was among them to greet me on my return—the partners, the staff and later on, the patients. They thanked me, ironically, for the single postcard now stuck derisively on the staffroom door. The computer had, it appeared, taken long service too, so long in fact that a new one now exchanged electronic discourtesies with its predecessor, side-by-side on the reception desk. The telephone came out in sympathy and there was a slim grey replacement studded with buttons and little lights, filled with discreet warbles and, rumour had it, piped music. The end-of-year balance that I had shrewdly planned to miss still wobbled uncertainly and the pile of out-of-date journals and long-past invitations tottered waist-high in the corner.

It took a little while to re-integrate. I had a tendency to offer lira in place of genuine Aussie money and a strange disinclination to read the papers, even the sports page, which increased the sense of social separation. I had a tendency to reminisce, which was promptly suppressed by watchful friends, to offer photographs, which were soon abandoned since each provoked an argument as to its time and place, and the opening gambit 'When we were in Barcelona' tended to engender groans. We eventually ran out of 'This time last week/month, we were menaced by Roman taxi drivers/overcharged by Spanish knife grinders/sneered at by English head waiters', and talked about local things.

I adjusted my neck to the unaccustomed necktie, entered into my diary the clinical obligations incurred while I was away, and went reluctantly back to work.

I don't know which was worse, the problems the locum had solved (and they were many and long overdue for it), or the ones he hadn't (and they too were many and alas unchanged). But I enjoyed the casual meetings in the street again, my street, if only to try Barcelona on some unwary acquaintance. It was good to rest my eyes again on green hills and empty car parks and I enjoyed the open cheerful approach, the straightforward comments, the ease of life in the Antipodes.

I cannot say that I romped with fresh zest through my work. There were so many coughs and colds (for it was winter time), so many sickies, so many maddening interrogatories from insurance companies and here and there a pneumonia to cure, a deathbed to attend to, a wound to stitch or a limb to plaster, to bolster my feeling of worth.

I'm nearly settled now, ploughing through the day's demands with a reawakened self-importance, offering opinions on local politics, beginning to believe again that I do write 'very interesting and helpful' letters of referral.

After three months and twenty thousand miles or more I guess there have been changes in me, if not in what I do. But now I'm back in general practice.

Small change.

more than a month of sundays

Even the most dedicated will admit to a certain melancholy on the Friday evening of a duty weekend. There is a faint but unexpressed feeling of grievance, a whiff of paranoia, an irrational jealousy of your partners, an unjustified aura of victimisation.

They, curse them, chat cheerfully about foreshadowed delights and, like the patients, leave the vital bit until last.

'Oh, by the way', they murmur over a departing shoulder, 'you might just hear from so and so'. And they leave with an uncompleted and impending saga of clinical or social catastrophe and the cold comfort of 'It's all in the notes'.

You grudgingly deny yourself the customary celebratory drink that marks the end of the working week and spend the evening one eye on the television, one ear cocked for the telephone, fielding from time to time the queries and requests that flow in once the surgery doors are shut. Always, it seems, from other people's patients.

By Saturday morning you are to some extent reconciled to work, while others saunter down the street and drop in for a repeat prescription or an ear syringing postponed from the working week.

You battle with a sense of irritation at the trivial and dismay at the serious problems that present, and confirm unhappily that it wasn't all in the notes. Only an illusory sense of martyrdom and devotion sustain you through the rest of the day.

By some inverse logic, the slack weekend is the worst. When the problems pile up, the telephones ring, calls beget calls, when the hospital is full, or claims to be, the ambulances are out on other jobs and the consultants have dwindled to unhelpful recorded messages, the whole thing becomes a challenge.

'All right', you say to some demon of medical confusion, 'what are you going to throw at me next?' and you set and revise priorities, cut your clinical coat to your chronological cloth and eat your long-delayed and thrice-warmed supper with a sense of achievement.

But when you're slack, a third patient arriving hot on the heels of the only two booked to see you or a single call in an otherwise empty afternoon is almost more than you can bear. If the telephone rings, you curse; if it doesn't, you start to worry lest the surgery answering machine is on the blink—again.

In the early years you worry that you will face some situation beyond your competence; later on, the realisation dawns that if you're not the best one you're the only one available. But the worry turns to other things, it never quite goes away.

You deal with the debris of afternoon sport—the ankles that might be broken, the noses that have been broken, the heads that might and might not be broken. You turn out to the stilted geniality of blood alcohol extractions, sew up the pot valiant, comfort the youngster who has swallowed mum's tablets in a fit of pique or wrecked dad's car and go eventually and wearily to bed. If there should be a telephone call through the night, it costs a glass of milk, a slice of cake and an hour before you go to bed again.

If there isn't, you wake to Sunday morning with a feeling you have scored.

Sunday morning for me is boiled eggs and proper coffee and relief that half the job is done. But Sundays are also the time for distant and slightly guilty relatives to swoop on neglected relatives and telephone the doctor to demand that something must be done. On Sundays the weekend nursing home staff discover lesions long-known and managed by the weekday crew, old ladies faint in church and bashful maidens from other towns come, boyfriend in tow, requesting HCGs.

By late afternoon you trifle with the thought that maybe it could wait until Monday and the usual doctor. You start to calculate just how many hours of bondage still remain. You wonder about your chances of seeing the Sunday serial and compile a list of clinical conundrums for your partners to solve next week. You turn on the alarm when you go to bed. The bell may toll for you on the morrow but, delicious thought, it will toll for them as well.

There is no sweeter sound than the radio that wakes you to the release of Monday morning, no finer sight than the clock that points to the hour of liberation.

What have you done? A bit of casualty—it takes a year or two in practice to understand the philosophical connection between 'casual' and 'casualty'—a bit of medicine, a certain amount of cursing, a fair bit of mooning around and a lot of reassurance.

You have held the fort, manned the bridge, raised the flag, earned a bit of money and spent a great deal of time. You have the weekend duty behind you and the happy prospect of leisure only five working days away.

Believe it or not, I like my job. I enjoy the unexpected wandering through the door and I appreciate (mostly) the unfathomable vagaries of humankind. I get a kick, sometimes in a painful place, from puzzles clinical and personal and marvel at the solutions that so often present unbidden, given time and patience.

In a faintly masochistic way I don't mind weekend duty.

But never on a Sunday.

———————— but am i right?

because it's there
a question of responsibility
signs for all times
who says?
advice and consent
good grief
here at the gate
the middle ground
the impotent doctor
shocks and starts
talking shop
supermarket medicine
a view from the sticks
quality street
on second thoughts
a plague on all our houses

because it's there

It was the end of a hot summer afternoon, a memorable day in this uncertain season, when the telephone call came in. I postponed that first inviting drink of the day and dropped in on my way home. I found a brawny youth of 18 summers, all better than the current one. He was red-haired and well-muscled, currently pale and, not surprisingly since he was in the shower at the time, rather damp.

His brother and I heaved him back to bed and I sat down to elicit a history. He had fainted. Now restored to something like normality, his story was graphic and uncomplicated, his diagnosis terse and, in my view anyway, accurate. He was, he said, 'B——-d'. The best I could do was to substitute a Latin label for his vigorous Anglo-Saxon.

I had delivered him as a baby and his mother reminded me of a similar episode in his late school days. I later confirmed in my notes the same pattern and the same clinical findings—slightly dilated pupils, and nothing else. I had not recorded his diagnosis on that occasion, but I guess he had used the same verb. It was a progressive school. I predicted the same complete and uncomplicated overnight recovery and left promising to review him on the next day, adding a vague and hazy suggestion of further investigation.

On reflection, that was perhaps a mistake. No doubt further inquiry and examination would offer nothing new and I would be stuck with a healthy, happy-go-lucky young man reduced to an introspective wreck by ill-considered investigation in the best scientific tradition.

A few years ago the question would never have arisen. There is a brand of men (and it is mostly men), beefy and muscular, who wade without a quiver into the toughest bar room brawl, who can swing a hammer I can hardly lift and lift a burden I can scarcely grasp, and whose imagination is only direfully excited by the sight of blood or the threat of injection. They fear nothing but the needle, no living being but the dentist.

You could pick them out on those parades when hapless servicemen lined up for their jabs. In those barbarous days you climbed over each pallid hulk and moved on to the next, while weedy, bespectacled medical orderlies discretely sniggered. My patient was such a man, toughened by hard work, hardened by tough sport. He could command everything but his autonomic nervous system.

But could it have been an odd epileptic variant, a singular metabolic quirk, and a lurking leash of capillaries where no capillaries should be? Would it not be wise or politic to order a CAT scan? I had only to lift the telephone, a scribbled form would command an EEG, the merest needle puncture would lay bare his innermost chemistry (and incidentally, repeat the original clinical picture)—it was all so readily to hand. Should I not, in fact, use it simply because it was there? It cost me nothing to arrange, the taxpayer would shoulder the bulk of the expense and the patient would bear the brunt of the fearsome venipuncture and the awesome entombment in the machine.

Then I realised that I was another victim of a new and potent syndrome sweeping through my colleagues like the Spanish flu.

I call it the Mallory-Everest syndrome. Apart from the fact that both can make you bloody sick, it bears no resemblance to the Mallory-Weiss syndrome. My Mallory was a mountaineer (of the 1930s I think), who when asked why he was so determined to climb Everest replied, 'Because it is there'.

And that, so help me, is what's happening to us. Why do a CAT scan, a battery of biochemical irrelevancies, an MRI or a profile of this, a screen of that? Because they are there. Not to clinch a diagnosis, monitor a treatment or detect a potential danger in a treatable phase, but because they are there. Because some hostile or supercilious colleague, some well-briefed lawyer, some penny-a-liner from the dailies, some investigator from prime time TV, will tell you that they are there, and will pillory you for daring to rely on your own clinical judgment, to trust your own observation, have faith in your own experience and believe in your own ability.

Only your friendly governmental counsellor—the one who's 'only here to help you doctor'—will applaud your restraint and remind you when you overspend.

When you think about it, that little room in which you spend so much of your working life is chock-a-block with unseen advisers. You face a patient sandwiched between a consumer affairs adviser at one elbow and a magazine doctor at the other; while a medical defence employee murmurs caution in one ear and a bureaucrat whispers parsimony in the other. In one corner behind you, the voice of postgraduate education poses questions, while from the other academic answers thunder forth. Educators, counsellors, public health advisers with messages to give, professors of prevention with barrows to push, they're all there, posturing for public attention, agreed only on one topic: the ignorance and inertia of people like you.

With so much attention, so much gratuitous advice, so many panaceas, it's a wonder the patient should need to consult you at all.

It's because, my friend, you're there.

a question of responsibility

About a month ago I received a telephone call mid-afternoon, inviting me to visit a lady who it appeared was tired, generally out of sorts and, this was the clincher, suffering from chest pain. A note appended to the details in the call book said it was not urgent.

Or was it? We have been conditioned to respond, like Pavlov's salivating dogs, to the faintest rumour of chest pain, to seize the bag and gallop, to exhibit aspirin and Morphia and the coronary preventive of the day, to rummage around for a cannula before it is seized from your hand by an expert paramedic. Later, should time and opportunity permit, you can take a hasty history and even a sketchy clinical examination before your patient is wheeled away to an ICU.

This patient was unknown to me, a recent arrival in what used to be a nursing home and is now a hostel (within the meaning of the Act). A place, that is, where 'clients' exercise their right of choice by refusing medical advice and forgetting essential medication. I knew at least that this lady had a husband who I had met, and who was elderly but fully competent and healthy for his 80 or so years. She too was elderly.

I went more or less straight away and met her. She was fully dressed, pale of face and obviously frightened, equally obviously determined not to make a fuss and conversant with, but not fluent in, the English language. The pain she talked of was not typical—it seldom is; hard clinical signs were not on view—they hardly ever are; and I found myself drying my hands in the minute and spotless bathroom wondering, not for the first time in nearly 40 years of clinical medicine, what the hell I was going to say, let alone do.

In one sense it was no problem. She might have, or might be about to have, an infarct. The elaborate apparatus geared for this eventuality only required a telephone call to be put in motion. She would fit, or would be forced to fit, into a predetermined protocol. She would be whisked off with cheery competence and unhesitating confidence, line in vein, electrodes on chest, triaged passed waiting casualties to a place filled with the beep of monitors and the swish of curtains nearly long enough to go around an almost comfortable bed. I could then go back to work filled with the satisfaction of a job well and easily done and later perhaps, a commendatory word from the medical registrar.

And what then? My patient might reappear in a day or two with five day's worth of aspirin in a paper bag, a low cholesterol diet sheet, an outpatient appointment and an ineradicable conviction that her life was hanging by a thread. Or she might have succumbed either to the severity of the illness or the necessary rigours of the treatment, simply because her time had come. She was 82, after all.

So I gave her Morphia, her husband my home telephone number and myself a sleepless night waiting for the telephone to ring and cursed my foolhardiness. Next morning I was greeted by a cheerful husband, a slightly narcotised but symptom-free wife and a wholly undeserved commendation for starting my day so early and being so attentive. Later on I confirmed the non-event with a normal ECG and unexceptionable enzymes. The stable door was firmly bolted but the steed, thank God, was still within.

Had she died, I would have been responsible and perhaps rightly called to account. But I was responsible anyway. As I am for every thing I do or don't do in my work. So are you and so is any professional who lives by advising others and takes on their problems. It is a conscious decision and the proper verb is 'take'. Nobody asked me to spend sleep and peace of mind on a dilemma I could have passed on to others without reproach.

No young primigravida knew what it cost me when her first stage was prolonged, or counted the times I balanced intervention against patience or retreat. I didn't have to do it and increasingly more I am not expected or even supposed to do it. I don't have to worry whether that wheezy child will worsen through the night, that frustrated teenager will make a realistic attempt on her life next time, or that histrionic headache signals a haemorrhage, hidden or impending.

But this is what we offer for sale. Every item that goes out of our shop is wrapped in a little bit of ourselves.

It isn't only the clinical decisions that keep you awake. For the most part, they're usually clear enough and even enjoyable. And when you are at a loss there are plenty of better-instructed colleagues eager to take them on. They have the added advantage of impartiality. They do not need to concern themselves with the social strands, the domestic factors or the maddening idiosyncrasies that we ignore at our peril.

This is not to disparage the specialist(s), but rather it is to value them at their true worth. They speak with an authority that I can never command. An outsider sees more of the game, and the shrewd and experienced observer perceives a whole that we the muddied umpires never raise our eyes to. They even include the GP-factor in the equation they are asked to solve.

A week or two later I was summoned at midnight by a calm but obviously stressed mother. She thought her 11-week's pregnant daughter had lost her baby.

'Can you be quick', she said, 'it's a bit of a mess'.

She had lost the baby and it was a mess clinically, emotionally and physically, but from my point of view it was a very simple one. This had happened, that must done and in such an order. It demanded nothing more than the application of skills learnt in professional adolescence—a protocol, in fact. It gave me a wry smile to hear the ambulance officer trying to extract from my patient a minute description of the pain she had suffered before the event and after the ergometrine. Had it been chest pain he would have been on more familiar ground and would not, I think, have been so particular. But he and his colleague took her away, which is what they were there for, and the whole unhappy business was tidied up. Later no doubt, there would be grief to comfort and surmount and perhaps anaemia to correct.

I went home and slept like a baby.

No, it is not the clinical problems that age us, but the setting and the people that bring them to us.

'You're the doctor', they say and they slip their load onto our aching backs, making us responsible. The best, the most dedicated, are sometimes tempted to pass them on. Tempted to send to a clinical psychologist (when an appointment becomes available) problems that need only time and patience to resolve; to ask a physician to say what they know and dare not say themselves—'There's nothing wrong with you'; to dump a frightened old lady's indigestion into a cardiac bed.

It's easy enough to understand why we all duck out from time to time. But why not all the time?

It's a question of responsibility.

signs for all times

One of the minor penalties of life in Tasmania is that drug detailers descend on us in groups. (I've searched in vain for a collective noun for them: a drone? a clutch? a bolus?) But, since many of the companies see us as a colonial appendage of Victoria, cut off by wind and tide and sometimes industrial action from this season's antibiotics and today's side-effect-free anti-histamines, they send them in batches to fill the waiting room at lunchtime and clog the car park with Commodores. For a day or so the samples pile up on the shelves and the brochures—too expensive to throw away and too glossy to recycle to humbler uses—encumber the desk, and the scribble pads and ballpoint pens are gratefully carted home.

One of their nicer habits is to invite us out to dinner. Every now and then a new product or a threatened old one whose sales are slipping will draw a hungry group of local doctors, united only by the prospect of a free meal, to see a videotape and hear an expert between the soup and the fillet steak. Sometimes, when the drug is expensive enough, they fly in Stars from Collins Street to talk physiology before the appetisers and tax evasion with the coffee, but mostly they rely on city colleagues we have seen before.

Most experts, to do them credit, make a point of failing to mention the product so lavishly advertised around the walls and we drive home heavy with the sponsor's hospitality, our integrity unbesmirched.

The last dinner I attended was addressed by a local cardiologist, a man whose modesty belies mastery of his subject and quiet skill with his patients. It is into his hands that I intend to place my ravaged coronaries after years of ignoring his advice. Need I say more?

He was talking about recent advances in the field and I went, not only because it saved on cooking at home, but because I hoped to understand what these echoes were that determined the fate of my patients and when a thallium scan would help. I'm sure he talked about all those things and I'm almost certain that given time I could have orientated those streaky snapshots, for all the world like weather maps, into recognisable valves and ventricles. But what I carried away I treasure even more.

He talked about taking histories. He suggested that the diagnosis of angina is a matter of history, of asking the right questions and drawing the right conclusions.

He talked about signs. He told us to feel for the apex beat, to gauge the quality of the pulse, to listen for and to the murmurs of a failing heart.

He talked, and it was a favourite phrase, of thinking. About the patient, the condition, the choices and the implications. He invited us, in other words, to go back to basics, to use eyes and ears and hands—and head.

And I realised with a pang of conscience how often I have ignored that message. How often I have been content simply to follow a well-worn track to an unreal destination. How often I have failed to check what I was told against what I could see, to reconcile what can be done with what should be done, to check the text beside me with the patient in front of me.

How cheap the equipment of a good clinician is, and how precious. What remains for any of us of our basic training? A few aphorisms perhaps, some models of how things are supposed to work and snapshots. There is an inborn textbook with some well-thumbed chapters that will open without conscious effort, but others are closed more or less for ever. Chiefly, it's little episodes—a rash, a lump or a noise—that remain with you as fresh as the day you first met them and with them the excitement that is the thrill of medicine.

Some years ago our practice was invited to take groups of students for a half-day session. We were free to show them anything we pleased. Show, not teach. So we scoured the practice for clinical signs and talked about them. We could have invited them to witness consulting techniques or held meaningful discussions on psychsomatics. We could have lectured at length on family dynamics until they nodded off. All of which are necessary parts of general practice, of course, and more significantly, subjects we could expound from the unshakeable pulpit of practical experience. But instead, we chose hisses and lumps and bumps. We threw ourselves open to contradiction. What student would refuse an argument where both sides start equal? We put our guests on an equal footing, not only with ourselves but with every preceding generation. The splash of obstruction sounds as loud in our ears as it does in Hippocrates'. And in doing so we caught their interest and rekindled our own.

It's one of the oddities of medicine that when the public say *clinical* they imply something coldly objective, scientifically inhuman. But we mean the reverse: it is the personal side of things, the idiosyncratic, even the intuitive.

I'm used to being a doctor. I'm proud of being a general practitioner, but what I value most of all is to be a clinician. This is what links me to all my colleagues and enables me to claim kinship with the Stars and acknowledge it with the tyros.

That was the simple message that I drove 15 miles to hear and brought my respected teacher 18 miles to give.

I wonder what the new drug was?

who says?

For those too serious for comic strips I should explain that there is a degenerate tribe of Red Indians whose exploits in and around the tiny town of Grimy Gulch are daily pictured in the Melbourne *Age* and other newspapers.

There is a Chief, an androgynous heir and, of course, a Medicine Man who makes occasional appearances. Now treating the dreaded Pepper Pox, a plague so deadly that the rash spreads to cover the very teepee walls, now binding the wounds of some battered brave and, in my favourite strip, conducting a typical consultation.

'What's your trouble?'

'I have an arrow in my back', and so he has for every reader to see.

'Show me your tongue.' Pause for total diagnosis and clinical decision making.

'Yes you have.'

To me it epitomises the experienced doctor at work. It is not sufficient to take the patient's word to acknowledge the lesion so strikingly displayed. There must be some little ritual magic, some awesome technical display before you set your professional seal on the blindingly obvious.

That, of course, is how it was. Now there would be deep and meaningful interchange, shrewd inquiries about smoking habits, pointed mention of cholesterol, inward speculation as to why that spitted sufferer really came. And how many venepunctures, how many scans with and without thallium, how many visits to respiratory physicians before the hapless victim is transported, face down, oxygen masked, IV-lined and plastered with sticky discs to find out how he feels, to the thoracic surgeon?

Or take Dr Watson, my beau ideal of late Victorian clinical certitude. Here he is in one of those casual, social consultations that makes every cocktail party a nightmare for the reluctantly confessed practitioner.

'A Doctor, eh?' cried he, much excited. 'Have you your stethoscope with you by any chance? I have grave fears as to my mitral valve. The aortic I know I can rely on but I should value your opinion upon the mitral.'
I listened to his heart as requested but was unable to find anything amiss.
'It appears to be normal.' I said. 'You have no cause for uneasiness.'
'I have long had suspicions as to that valve. I am delighted to hear they are unfounded.' [2]

Can you imagine a modern cardiologist, let alone a GP, so rash as to make that Olympian assessment without so much as a chest X-ray? Can you imagine a patient trusting enough to believe him or a lawyer disinterested enough to let him get away with it?

First we casually pulled down an eyelid and prescribed an iron tonic. Then we pricked a finger, fiddled with coal gas or a Sahli wedge and ordered iron tablets. Now we send away an FBE, perhaps serum for iron studies, a little plastic pot of faeces, even invite some whitecoat to suck marrow from the very bones and only when the last report is in, the dread implications outlined and dismissed, do we send him trembling to the chemist.

What is a broken rib? A hell of a pain in the chest that cuts your breath after you fell over, a tender spot on the chest wall and a grunt of protest on rib compression—or a shadow on a photograph?

'Ah but', you say, 'what about a pneumothorax?' You need a chest X-ray for that, a wholly different matter. Will you order both?

'And what about the legal implications?' you reply.

What about them? Will your picture make a ha'p'orth of difference to your treatment—or lack of it?

You should, you must investigate if it's germane to the diagnosis—or lack of it. You may well perform a test on your patient's reasonable request. You might obey your professors when they advise that this or that investigation is (lovely word) mandatory—at least until you are far enough away in time and long enough away in experience to think for yourself. But you must not let lawyers make your clinical decisions for you.

I wonder how many gallons of sterile urine deluge the laboratories daily and what influence the inevitably negative reports have on those who pass them. One can so easily drift into using investigations to cover indecision, to postpone, evade and finally ignore the judgment you have been paid to make. To pass the buck (I nearly wrote buckie) to the radiologist, the autoanalyser, the tired technician glancing wearily at yet another normal film.

'Ring up next week', you say. 'I'll let you know the results.' And a week later an anxious patient learns from you, or your receptionist, that 'they're all normal'. Where does that leave a pain not described in the textbooks, a bizarre episode of instability, a rash that comes and goes and comes again? Everything is normal it seems—except the patient. Who is reassured by normal findings in abnormal feelings? Only the doctor.

There is a no less uncomfortable parallel for us too. Who has not turned up an unexpected abnormality in an ostensibly healthy patient? One that begs the question but conceals the answer or answers the question that was never asked. Do I tell, and cover the revelation with meaningless reassurance or embark on a fruitless quest for some non-existent malady that ends with loss of face, loss of temper and loss of patient to a wiser colleague. Or do I keep quiet and maybe set an ambush for myself somewhere down the track.

We can't escape the relentless march of technological advance, sideways as it sometimes seems to be, no more than we can hide behind the authority of the anonymous expert. We cannot pauperise the nation to cover our clinical inadequacies. We sometimes have to make the judgment, choose the option, say the word.

Who says?

I says.

advice and consent

I've forgotten which of our mentors it was, so many years ago, who said to us in all sincerity: 'Never give advice unless you are paid for it and if possible, never give advice at all.'

Strange comment to make to those who were about to earn their bread and butter by that very means.

As to the first part there can be no argument. What is given for nothing is valued at nothing. Part of the mystique and success of specialisation is just that. The advice tendered may be exactly the same as yours and mine but since it is more expensive it carries greater weight. Even the doctors who fill the back pages of the weeklies are paid for what they say about blackheads, plastic surgery or PMT. Even the comments from the Chair—Faculty, College or Foundation—are paid for, in media attention and strident misreporting. Even those who studiously avoid commitment, offer a range of options, a choice of avenues, a modest openness of mind, are credited with God-like prescience or megalomaniacal certitude.

A strangled grunt can be interpreted as a life-long interdiction of, say, tomatoes: 'He said it's poison to you, all that acid.'

Or doom-laden prophesy: 'They only gave me three months [oh, generous they] and that was 10 years ago.'

Or a definitive diagnosis: 'Almost on the verge of a nervous breakdown, those were his very words.'

Only when you go to the trouble of explaining in wearisome detail, paint the picture with elaborate brush strokes, outline each separate remotely possible consequence and offer sincere and soundly-based strategies to secure or circumvent them, only then are your efforts subsequently dismissed with the stinging phrase: 'He [or more commonly they] never told me a thing.'

As increasingly we take cover in conditional clauses, wallow in ifs and buts, hedge our bets, clear our yardarms and cover our bases, so the demand for informed consent grows.

There were, and you still meet them occasionally, those who are just too compliant. 'You're the doctor' is the phrase that you learn to interpret as: 'You know everything, and can do what you like with me. But, if you don't get it right you'll be hearing from my solicitors.'

There are those who approach from the opposite corner—and believe that you are by definition, ignorant, rapacious and ludicrously incompetent. There are those who ask searching questions and dispute the answers, demand drugs without side effects, surgery without the possibility of mishap and cure without inconvenience.

Young mothers seek unnecessary antibiotics for their snotty children or reject them on those rare occasions when at least in your judgment they are really needed. But judgment is a word that has changed sides in the consulting room. Once it stood for an informed choice by the doctor, now it implies a hostile appraisal by the patient. It's like that other bogy word 'discrimination'. Where it once meant discernment and appropriate selection, it now signifies and reproves any hint of distinction between humankind whether by gene, environment or choice.

Young mothers-to-be worry about the possible effects of drugs on their unborn child, and so they should, but so does their doctor. Their doctor will not knowingly hazard two lives for the want of proper information. I understand and applaud the concern, but could I not be given credit for sharing it?

Life presents us all with cruel choices sometimes and when it has to do with health and wellbeing, what can or can't be cured, what must or need not be endured, then we are professionally involved. It is a costly business for all parties, not cash but fear and ignorance, not income but knowledge and compassion. It took me many years to learn that any problem is by definition soluble. What is insoluble is not a problem, but a condition beyond your power to change except by adaptation.

The advice we offer for sale depends on our knowledge of options and possible outcomes, a reasonably accurate estimation of odds and a fair appreciation of the personal cost to life and living.

In the matter of chances and whatever else makes up the neglected art of prognosis, you can only offer a percentage, a fraction, knowing that however high the denominator, the numerator is only one—the one facing you across the desk. One person and one question. And only time knows the answer to it.

But there is another part of the cost equation and it is in assessing this that we are most likely to come to grief.

What to say and how to say it. And how much to tell and how much to gloss over or postpone.

Tell them everything, of course, you say, but 'everything' implies that the anxious listener has a working knowledge of structure and function and the composure to put it to the test with a distracted and a disturbed body. And at a time when, to the catalogue of technical questions, however expertly answered, there is another inner list: What about the family? The firm? The future? Will there be pain and if so, how much? How long will it last? Will I ever be myself again? And hardest of all to answer—why me?

And you? You have to pick your words carefully and find comfortable phrases for cruel realities. How do you break anything gently? Add to this a realisation of urgency and necessity, some previous experience—often, as it turns out, misleading—of your patient's capacity to bear and understand and a simultaneous internal translation of your language to his or hers, or both. You have to steer a course between brutal truth and soothing generality, you have to be accurate without alarming, and encourage but not minimise. You cannot send your patient to the theatre blind from ignorance—or terror.

And now to add to that perplexity, somewhere in the corner of your mind a supercilious advocate makes scornful comment on your best endeavours.

I do give advice and charge for it and am sometimes paid in gratitude more durable than coin. I do seek informed consent in terms that vary with every individual that needs it. I'm paid for that too and I too bear a cost.

I sometimes wonder which is greater.

good grief

'It takes three to make quarrels. There is needed a peace maker. The full potentialities of human fury cannot be reached until a friend of both parties tactfully intervenes'.[3]

It is with this laudable intention that I entered a debate on 'Learning to cope with grief' in the columns of a distinguished medical journal. I could not, of course, claim to be a friend of any of the parties, although with a bit of luck I ended up the sworn enemy of all.

I think the phrase that really got me was: 'We [i.e. the doctors] can also show our feelings, for example crying, as a gesture of support, without shame as this is quite natural and an obvious display of our caring.'

Now I rarely cry these days (although I don't mind quiche), but if and when I have, it has been when some tragedy has robbed me of any other response. Grief, anger, despair or guilt sometimes seek physical relief and happy are they that can vent it without harm to others or destruction to themselves. Happier still are those who can use it to widen their understanding of themselves and their sympathy for others.

I certainly would not quarrel with such authorities as Mal McKissock or Beverly Raphael who have discovered what most of my patients have stumbled on for themselves: 'He or she has got to have his or her cry out'. Sooner or later they do. What puzzles me is the suggestion of crying as a means of condolence, 'a gesture of support', a professional response, an instant black armband, a decorous black handkerchief covering dry eyes.

There are patients whose death, for one reason or another, strikes with a tragic personal pang, and there are mourners whose grief wakens a painful echo in ourselves. It may be that I too am moved to tears that I cannot and perhaps should not withhold. But I cry from grief, even from sympathy, but never as a gesture of support.

Empathy is a word that always troubles me. The dictionary defines it as 'mentally entering into the feeling or spirit of another person'. As a spiritual exercise it is no doubt superb. It teaches humility, enlarges understanding and engenders charity. But, by its very nature, where it enlightens it can also darken. In opening the doors to another's mind you slam them on your own. If you would truly share another's thoughts and feelings you must renounce your own.

So as the doctor, summoned to a distraught widow, a circle of agitated relatives and an anxious priest, you are there because you have been called to a situation, which, to the participants at least, is out of control. You will need all your resources and professional skill no less than human understanding. You must be detached but involved, strong but gentle, if you are to do your job.

You alone in that distracted company are expected to act. You alone are looked to for guidance, appealed to for help. You cannot answer those appeals with muffled sobs or dodge behind your handkerchief. You know—who does not—that grief must work and tears must flow. You know too, that there is a point at which endless lamentation is self-defeating. Even the overwrought must rest, and sleep however bought can set a limit to the keenest agony of loss. It is your professional judgment that is needed and tested by each consistently different occasion—when to ventilate and when to abridge.

There is a lady in our practice who through the years repaid our services with chocolate eclairs and creamy layer cakes. One day she brought her husband to me en route for major surgery. She didn't think he was fit for it and, after examination, neither did I. The anaesthetist to whom I confided my misgivings was suavely reassuring, but later the next evening I got a message that God had sided with me.

As I approached the house of mourning I could hear the new widow screaming amidst a confused medley of expostulations and breaking crockery. I was let in by an alarmed relative and for the next 10 minutes I pursued my patient through the house, pleading, cajoling and exhorting until, with trembling hands but dry eyes, I penned her in a corner and gave her not condolences but Largactil, and she eventually subsided.

The next morning she greeted me at the door, tear-worn but tranquil.

'How are you?' I asked.

'Oh, I've had my cry—I'm all right now. Would you like a cup of tea?'

We sat together and talked about her husband, about her loss and her—to me—well-founded anger at his professional advisers, until she talked herself out and said 'I'd better let you go'.

She doesn't often come to the surgery, she doesn't often need to these days, but she still brings in the cakes.

here at the gate

It's one of the commoner cliches that describe and even congratulate us as the gatekeepers to the health care system. There we stand, directing and controlling a flow of acquiescent patients—this one to intensive care, that one to the rheumatologist, this little fellow needs guidance, that ancient dame Meals on Wheels. Just step this way.

But it isn't like that at all really, is it? The determined patient denied their third or fourth opinion, or as many more as it may take until it coincides with their own, will get one down the road. The asthmatic presenting himself to Casualty is entangled in a mesh of assessment and expert evaluation, counselling and breathing classes—mostly by nurses—that involves his own (hollow possessive) doctor at most in writing repeat prescriptions and countersigning the social worker's requisition for a nebuliser. The casual dropper-in to a cardiac risk shop will indeed be returned to his doctor—for a referral to a cardiologist.

More and more it seems to this jaundiced gatekeeper, an application for home nursing must first pass the scrutiny of a supervisor and is regarded more as a basis for discussion than a stimulus to action. Junior residents sit in judgment on requests for urgent admission from their lowly colleagues in the field.

In passing, I was fascinated by a recent locally researched article that showed that 40 something per cent of requests for urgent admission to the teaching hospital by GPs were accepted—or should that read 'granted'. There was an air of modest congratulation that nearly half the time the outside (the adjective is chosen advisedly) doctor was right—at least by the standards of the hospital. No mention was made of the hospital's criteria or, impious thought, how often they were wrong. We were gently reprimanded for failing to detail the social history so instantly available at 3 a.m. and so essential in medical emergencies or providing (fair enough) a medication list (I am chary of sending the actual medication as it will be (a) confiscated and (b) changed anyway), and softly slapped (fairer still) on the grounds of legibility. But typewriters are not that portable.

When, I wondered, will we see the companion study, tabulating how often the letters receive a timely answer, or in fact any answer at all? Did the interim discharge summary—the third, fading carbon copy of a bald handwritten list of abbreviations—reach the doctor before the undertaker? It happens sometimes, even in teaching hospitals. When, on average, did two pages of no longer relevant biochemistry, a terse paragraph of completed procedures and a list of generic medications signed by a stranger arrive to signal the end of the episode? How often did the consultant under whose name these compositions appear ever look at them and how did they compare in speed and value with his own professional correspondence?

But back to the gate. It has become an accepted axiom that health is too important to be left to doctors, particularly GPs. Six years of medical school, three or four years vocational training and unlimited enrolment at the school of hard knocks and bitter experiences don't equate with a three-year stint in a College of Nursing, a degree in Sociology or a couple of courses in Family Planning. Our local health board's five-year plan squeezed in two brief references to general practice in 180 pages of health promotion, staff development and client satisfaction.

Take nursing homes. Admission now depends on the permission of a team—two nurses and one social worker—applying cast iron rules ('guidelines') designed to save the government money, as inflexible in application as they are unrealistic in practice. A distant and sympathetic bureaucrat countersigns. Half way down the two-page application form a little block is provided for the family doctor to record pathological diagnosis and pharmaceutical treatment. The system is palliated by the good sense and fair-mindedness of those who administer it, but inevitably over the years they have passed from assessment to influence to absolute control. The gate is locked and the gatekeeper left voiceless on the other side.

In an egalitarian age, when to be in the minority is ipso facto to be privileged, entitled to more care, more money, more misdirected assistance than the rest, there is, paradoxically, more division in an already divided society. Instead of levelling the ghettos we are building bigger more luxurious ones. An excluded group becomes exclusive. The gates are locked on the other side.

We mustn't be part of this. Health is one and indivisible—it is not restricted to a single section of the population. We take on all comers on a basis of need (not want), even if the subject is white, middle class and of English descent. The absence of Aboriginal blood does not exclude anyone from their health care and the possession of a Y chromosome does not exclude anyone from women's health issues, any more than a preference for sports medicine excuses ignorance of sexually transmitted disease. An aptitude for minor surgery does not absolve you from the care of the dying or those who mourn their passing. Carried to its logical conclusion, the opposite view assigns paediatrics exclusively to infantile clinicians, psychiatry, if it is not already, to mad doctors. The result, like the specialties, is childish—and mad.

We are not gatekeepers. How can we be when there are so many gaps in the fence on either side? We are stretcher bearers, wandering over the battlefield looking at wounds, not uniforms; patching where we can with what we have to hand; offering the assurance of seasoned if limited skill, the security of dispassionate competence and the comfort of good intent. Picking up this man, that woman, these children, as gently as we can and carrying them to the proper place. For if our skill is limited we know, who better, the limitations of our colleagues. Where we falter in depth they may fail in scope. However swift the recovery, however expert the attention on the way, it must be pointless if you don't know where to go. And we're rather good at that.

'Come into the garden, Maud', sang Tennyson and a thousand tenors after him. 'I am here at the gate alone.'

So are we.

the middle ground

For the last couple of years our little town has enjoyed the ministrations of an alternative medicine man. He is, like many of his successful confreres, medically qualified. So at least he knows something of the medicine he has turned his back on to graze the greener pastures of alfalfa, wheat germ and royal jelly where his orthodox colleagues cannot follow him. Lately, he is reported to be wavering between oriental religion and a therapy for terminal cancer involving self-administered coffee enemas (for the patient, that is) and intravenous ozone.

I know nothing of his medicine apart from his failures and he has, no doubt, exactly the same impression of mine. So any judgment of mine is rooted in ignorance, prejudice and perhaps derision. Neither a professional commitment to scientific objectivity nor a personal predilection for tomfoolery qualifies me to comment.

I do, I think, recognise an emphasis on the person rather than the pathology, which is increasingly permeating our own discipline. And I sometimes wonder if in pursuing this we may not lose sight of our essential obligation for accurate anatomical and pathological diagnosis and rational and objectively assessed treatment.

Then, a month later, another colleague called to introduce himself on the eve of setting up a pain clinic. He was, it appeared, an anaesthetist whose interest and skill in introducing local anaesthetics to the most obscure and recondite nooks had led him into this new venture. I certainly could not quibble at the minute anatomical accuracy and knowledge that his art demanded, nor question the laboratory pedigree of the complex chemicals at his disposal. He rather lost me after the endorphins (which I hitherto equated with scuba diving in covered swimming pools), but the message seemed to be that pain untouched by his manoeuvres didn't count.

So there it was. Since I am neither clever enough to insinuate a minuscule cannula into the greater superficial petrosal nor stupid enough to wash the whole thing out with Maxwell House, what the Hell am I (or for that matter you) here for?

The acute chest pain that you took an anxious pride in assessing and organising initial treatment for, is now whisked away by two uniformed quasi-cardiologists who brush you aside politely while conning the monitor, adjusting the oxygen and putting a line in. The acute belly ache, that diagnostic challenge and therapeutic poser, where there were signs for the careful to find and pointers for the shrewd to follow, is now the province of a peeping Tom with a light that goes round corners and a wire that sizzles the spot. The unstable diabetic, that life-long game of chess with move and counter move, now ambles in periodically for more reagent strips when the clinic is closed over the long weekend.

Other experts have shouldered our anxieties and the pride and responsibilities that went with them. Are we, the backbone of the profession as we like to think, being inexorably dissected by the pressures of new technology and the seduction of a specious philosophy?

Is there a need for anatomy when you can see the whole thing in 3-D on the video screen? Is it still acceptable to put together five clinical and one common sense and arrive at a conclusion without a nod from the pathologist or a nuclear medicine buff? Are we doomed to pursue only those biochemical abnormalities that the auto analyser detects in healthy people? Is the long catalogue of occasional triumphs and occasional disasters, the never-to-be forgotten intuitive flash, the always regretted and needless oversight that we call experience, of no value whatsoever?

If the future holds little more than routine check-ups, little chats on the evils of butter and tobacco, requests for needles and council houses and long interviews with the rejected clients of the social worker, there seems to be little point in the rigorous selection and arduous training now prescribed.

Surely there is a middle ground. A field where pathology meets personality and wise and wary doctors learn humility in applying the rigidity of science to the vagaries of humankind. Where well-trained and compassionate men and women strive to adapt and interpret, reconcile and support and use their clinical skill to enlarge their understanding and extend their tolerance to those that turn to them.

If we are threatened, and perhaps we always have been, our defence is in our own hands. We must come to terms with the new developments, select those that offer genuine benefit to us and our patients and adopt, adapt and use them. I can't believe that gastroscopy is all that difficult. I too can read a pathology report, especially if they put in the normal values for me. I have been known to put local anaesthetic in and around the brachial plexus, the pudendal nerve and a digital nerve or two. I'm not that bad with instant coffee, either.

Interview techniques, circumscribed psychotherapy with

defined and limited objectives and gentle ventilation of anguish or despair, do not really demand five year's understudying a shrink. It's all our ground.

The middle ground.

the impotent doctor

A few months ago I was consulted by a youngish man with an oldish problem. He was tired and irritable, troubled by palpitations at night and constant left-sided chest pain by day. He was restless and moody at home, bored and ineffectual at work.

'There must be something wrong with me', he said, 'Isn't there a tonic you could recommend?'

Examination convinced me (at least) that there wasn't and I knew that there isn't. While he dressed, I pondered the problems such a person presents. How far should you undertake expensive investigations in the usually fruitless pursuit of reassurance, and how do you convince the worried that their physical dreads are groundless but their worries real? How too are the worries unearthed and confronted?

It turned out that the basic problem was lack of confidence, severe enough to drive him out of the job that his diligence had gained, but his incompetence had lost him.

He was now, by a crowning irony, selling health foods from door to door. We talked for a while and I think I reached him. But what could I do for him? Psychotherapy? Maybe. Psychiatry? Probably not. Psychotropics? No way. In summary, I said that I didn't think that he was ill and I didn't think I could help, and diffidently suggested 'Grow', an organisation that addresses this problem in this area.

After he left I ruminated further about him and the common problem he exemplified.

What a field day for the moneymakers and alternative experts. How many courses of megavitamins, spinal manipulations, needles judiciously implanted, mantras monotonously repeated, might offer illusory and expensive relief?

I, the orthodox quack, sent him away, but there were half a dozen unlettered sages who would take him on—or in.

It is a paradox that the more orthodox medicine discovers, the less it is respected. Yesterday, it was a largely uninformed patient who submitted without question to a largely ignorant but didactic doctor. Today, a knowledgeable but defensive doctor labours to convince a half-informed and sceptical patient.

We have discarded the white coat, descended from the pedestal, abandoned all those comfortable panaceas—focal sepsis or constipation, dietary indiscretion or genetic disposition—and sat down to argue the pros and cons of this procedure, that drug, the other approach. Increasingly, we admit our uncertainty. And when we turn around to pick up the mantle it has gone; when we go to resume the platform it is occupied by someone else.

Our alternative opposition has collected our discarded enthusiasms, mounted the vacated pulpit and assumed an authority we no longer dare to claim.

We don't have all the answers—but they do.

The educated public who subject us to such relentless questioning on hysterectomies or home deliveries embrace with enthusiasm the larger lunacies of fringe medicine. The pregnant schoolmistress who refused ear syringing on the grounds that it might hurt her unborn baby, plastered herself with vitamin E cream, that prince of sensitisers.

It should take at least two surgeons to decide on an appendicectomy, but it takes only one naturopath to order twice-weekly colonic lavage.

I'm not embarking on a critique of alternative medicine, rather pointing out the logical difficulty it presents. If iridology is right, foot massage is plain stupid; if milk causes migraine, meditation is pointless and manipulation downright dangerous.

Not all the runners can win the medical Melbourne Cup. It could even be that top weight veteran Orthodoxy, although it's not the favourite any more.

What marks us out, perhaps, is the very uncertainty we now admit. Can *you* guarantee painless delivery, unfailing surgical success, drugs without side effects or treatment without hazard?

If you can't, you're one of us—a true professional.

shocks and starts

I was told this story quite recently, although the incident happened more than 15 years ago.

A father, the narrator, arrived home from the office one evening to find his wife pale but composed, ushering out the family doctor.

'Don't worry', she murmured, 'everything's under control. I'll tell you as we go upstairs.'

It appeared that their 14-year old son on his way home from school had been skylarking on the parapet of a railway bridge. In the course of his antics he threw a scarf belonging to a fellow scholar, a girl, on to the electrified tracks below. In a belated spirit of chivalry, or perhaps for fear of the consequences, he climbed down to rescue it. It was raining.

His foot slipped and 750 volts of outraged electricity chose him as an earth. Miraculously, the only result was a pair of molten sneakers, a scorched cheek and the fright of a lifetime.

Hence the summons for the local doctor, promptly answered, but unsupported by the first response unit, the back-up ambulance or an eager team of experts and hence, of course, the staircase bulletin.

The doctor, after summing things up, prescribed an emollient and a night's rest, but devoted most of his attention to the emulsified sneakers, as well he might, and left expressing his admiration of that particular brand. I think he could also have commended the mother, who had neither panicked nor magnified what must have been, in retrospect, an anguishing experience. She too was obviously of premium brand and first-class materials.

The boy himself, white where he was not singed, and as terrified as he was relieved, eventually settled down to a troubled rest, doubtless shared by his anxious parents. The doctor called again next day and pronounced his patient to be very lucky, very foolish and fit for school in a day or two. Later on his school friends sat around the bed and after a brief period of awed decorum joked and scuffled as schoolboys always do.

Over the next day or two the superficial marks faded but the patient remained listless and unsettled and the doctor was summoned again.

What did he do? He consulted neither psychiatrist nor psychologist, called in no counsellor, offered no sedative. He sat on the edge of the bed and as the boy's mother described it, 'tore one heck of a strip off' her son (his father had an even more vivid if terser description) and told him to get up and go back to school.

And so he did, that traumatised adolescent, and forgot all about it soon enough. Unless you count a successful career in advertising, he has suffered not a pennyworth of harm since.

When I heard that tale my admiration went out to that admirable GP.

First, that he had the courage of his scientific convictions that no long-term physical damage could result, that he did not hedge his bets with a prolonged convalescence to chronic invalidism, dodge his responsibilities by fruitless investigations or referral to a stranger to say what had to be said, or do what had to be done.

Second, that he did not foster a sense of psychological insecurity in patient and parents by a series of counselling sessions designed to make a heedless boy express fears he had not had time to feel, or allay anxieties which, if he even perceived, he was perfectly capable of allaying for himself.

Third, that his confidence in his own judgment rubbed off on parents and patient alike.

·I sometimes feel that a whole industry is now devoted to the management of stress, however that nebulous and inescapable factor is defined. It is assumed that anyone who suffers the shock of the unexpected, exposure to accidental hazard, has had a brush, however fleeting, with death or disaster, has witnessed or taken part in scenes of horror or suffered an assault on flesh or senses, is unequipped to deal with it without professional assistance.

'Let me through', says the fictional doctor, 'I'm a doctor'. (In real life we cower behind a lamp post until conscience or a conscientious spouse drags us to reluctant participation.)

Now it seems to be 'Let me through, I'm a counsellor' and spectators stand respectfully aside for them to stride to the psychological rescue.

I think of a mate who at 17 came ashore from his newly docked warship to sort through the debris of an air raid for the scattered fragments of the casualties. I think of my neighbour who, at much the same age, worked with the Dutch resistance hiding Jews whose fate, if detected, he would share. I think of an ex-partner who, by his wife's account, climbed nightly from his bed to issue fire orders learnt on the Normandy beachhead long after that war had ended; and of another colleague who spent weeks in an open boat in the Atlantic and lived to tell the tale—but never does. I think of patients who daily faced death by beating or sickness and slow starvation and came back to get on with their lives, hiding those honourable scars.

I think of generations of women surviving, or not, the hazards of primitive midwifery and the heartbreak of losing children so hardly borne. And I wonder what these unremarkable people did for counselling and consolation. Religious faith? Patriotic pride? Intestinal fortitude? Whatever it was, have we lost the knack of it?

I cannot deny that the mechanisms fail sometimes. We all see the consequences in our daily work. We all strive to support and prevent where we can. The wonder is that they work so well, so often. The skill is to know when to intervene and when to stand aside, when to open the door and when close it between what has been and what is now.

That doctor had it.

talking shop

She was a complete stranger to me. It was Easter Monday, I was characteristically disgruntled at having to work and she was hopping mad.

'I want an X-ray', she said.

I suppressed a number of equally tart rejoinders and restricted myself to offering her a chance to tell her tale from the beginning. It was simple enough: a sprained wrist (whatever that may be), five weeks ago, a doubtful diagnosis and a crepe bandage, a visit to casualty four weeks later, an X-ray, a fracture and an ill-applied plaster, which the applier refused to remove. Then she took the matter quite literally into her own hands, removed the plaster, bought a splint from the chemist and presented herself to me.

Whatever she might need, and it took a little while to work that out, there was no doubt what she wanted—blood. But I didn't see why it should be mine.

I flipped through a number of familiar roles. I listened (the doctor as confidant), I took the picture (the doctor as technician), I advised (the doctor as expert) and I charged her (the doctor as shopkeeper). It was, remember, a public holiday and I was on my own.

I declined, to my credit, to invite her to come back to me (the doctor as tout) or to criticise my colleagues (the doctor as ratbag), and she departed mollified if not satisfied, appreciative if not effusive.

She had got what she wanted and I had, I think, given her what she needed.

Happy the clinical encounter when the two coincide. This is the crux of consultation, reconciling your patient's demands with your professional conscience, dealing reasonably with the unreasonable, affably with the intemperate and making allowances for those who give none.

We are not supposed to be authoritarian any more, paternalism is out and uncles, even Dutch uncles, are eschewed. We must offer each hesitant suggestion on the assumption that six year's training and God knows how much bitter experience equates with high school biology (at best), the back pages of women's magazines and those scary little pamphlets that come with every bottle of pills. Only when the subject is salt, butter or nicotine can we, nay must we, pontificate and threaten (the doctor as governess).

All this has to be performed against a background of indignantly shuffling feet, reproachful coughs from the waiting room and a ringing telephone that sooner or later has to be answered.

It calls for a skill once described for me by an adept accountant. He called it 'satisficing', which may roughly be described as the art of keeping most of the customers happy most of the time; of giving sufficient time and attention to each as will send them away at least temporarily reassured.

The whole problem has become bedevilled by the advent of consumerism and the alleged benefits of competition. Alas in medicine, as in all endeavours constrained by reason and reality, the customer is not always right. Damaged human articles cannot always be repaired and can never be sent back to the maker or replaced. In our trade there are no guarantees from retailer or manufacturer.

How can you keep a shop where no goods are sold, where only one outcome is inevitable and such standards as there are, are comparative and subjective? In the clash between I want/you need, I feel/you are, what resolution is possible? Yet we try to do this every day. In physical things with some success. There should be chairs in a waiting room, there should be enough and they should be comfortable. Three levels of attainment which become more subjective as they ascend. What is comfortable? Your patient may sink his aching back into the cushions with gratitude, but he will not thank you when, at last, he tries to get up again. Need and want, it crops up everywhere.

It is the same with the intangibles. You should be available, but for how long and how often? Most people appreciate being able to telephone their doctor at will, except the one whose consultation is interrupted thus. Nobody likes to be kept waiting, but nobody cares to be dismissed with undue haste.

'My word doctor, you are busy today', says some thoughtful soul and settles in for half an hour of triviality, maddeningly prolonged with 'While I'm here' freckles and a routine Pap. We all accept the duty to give time where it is needed (not wanted); we are all criticised for saving it where it is not.

If you call my customers 'patients' I shall give them what they need, if you call them 'clients' I shall give them what they pay for and if you call them 'consumers' I shall give them what they want. According to the dictionary, a patient is 'one undergoing medical or surgical treatment', 'a sufferer' or, and I like this one, 'one enduring delay with calmness and equanimity'. Vain hope.

A client, on the other hand is 'one who employs or seeks advice from a professional adviser' and a consumer is simply 'one who consumes'—principally, I suspect, the professional adviser in question.

It is the consumer who flits from shop to shop in search of certificates or ever more expensive and usually toxic drugs, bigger and better investigations paid for by somebody else and seeks to replenish their bulging medicine chest from half a dozen competing sources. Those little coteries of the weekend migraine sufferer whose headaches only pethidine will relieve consume—and competition supplies. Competition builds 24-hour clinics and consumers throng them.

The only honest competition in our trade is, like golf, with oneself—the never-ending struggle with what one needs to know but doesn't, what one ought to do but can't and, like golf, there is a handicap, a human preference for occasional escape.

Like supermarkets or corner stores, open all hours or weekdays only, there comes a time to put up the shutters, bow out the last customer and shut the shop.

Until the next time.

supermarket medicine

For years now our practice management experts and accounting gurus have been disdainfully describing general practice as the last of the cottage industries and urging us to face our responsibilities as business people. Little by little, with a staff manual here, an accounting machine there, we have streamlined our bulky selves into something like a business mould. There have been gratifying economies in practice, expenses that have almost paid the leasing charges, extra stationery bills and escalating accounting fees. We can point with diffident pride at the record system, the cashbook and the computer bubbling in the corner. We have moved out of the cottage into the corner store.

Then, one day, we awoke to find a supermarket on the way if not yet across the street. That fellow—not a Fellow I believe—from the city moved in and the era of the one stop doc. shop was here and flourishing.

We were appalled.

How dare he spoil the brutes with umpteen comfortable chairs and no waiting, set his hours by their requirements, his service by their demands and his salaries by what the traffic would bear?

We could explain away the commercial success and predict impending collapse with relish, but not the popularity. Old Macdonald might have a farm, to say nothing of an ocean yacht and a Swiss bank account, but he had patients, many of them and mostly ours. What had become of our cherished assets: personal care, total commitment and 24-hour cover? No wonder we felt cheated and a little sad.

But at least that particular medical entrepreneur was medically qualified—one, up to a point, of our own. But maybe even that's not really necessary. There was to be a chain of clinics in Melbourne masterminded by a duo of laundry owners and real estate agents. It would be, we were told, slightly more austere, dare we say down market, but none the less would offer radiology, pathology, counselling and psychology in addition to one or two qualified doorpeople/secretaries to direct the traffic and take care of the paper work.

There is nothing particularly unholy in an alliance of business and medicine.

My alma mater was founded by a miserly but finally repentant bookseller who sold out of the South Sea Bubble before it burst and invested in good works while there was yet time. The outpatients bore the name of a successful hop merchant with a sideline as an impresario and the private wing represented the serial defeats on the golf course of a canny physician by a maker of motor cars. Even the newest student building was the gift of a supermarket magnate.

Patronage is one thing, but possession another. Will the professional staff of these enterprises, however highly paid, fringe benefitted or awarded a slice of the action, sometimes pine for the independence of thought, action and responsibility that the humble cottager buys with their overdraft? Will there be some corner of a foreign Kmart that is forever College?

Not for nothing are they called chain stores.

Action brings reaction. Already there is talk of pre-paid health care and season ticket medicine, and before long it will be capitation fees and subsidised mediocrity: service of a sort for all and satisfaction for none.

As far as I see it makes little difference whether your salary is paid by a department or a department store. Neither has a soul to be damned or a body to be kicked.

The new departures may be the best thing since sliced bread.

But I'd rather have a cottage loaf.

a view from the sticks

It's always nice to get a letter, even a critical one. At least someone out there has been sufficiently stirred to put keyboard to screen and pay me the compliment of rational opposition, as Jane Austen more or less put it.

Sometimes, when that nice man from Melbourne rang in search of copy and I faced a blank screen with an even blanker mind, then turned it off for a hundred specious reasons, I was tempted to dispatch an earlier offering in the hope that it would slip unnoticed into next month but one. In 20 years I had a few to choose from.

The less charitable might have suggested that I did indeed write the same one every time, the same quasi-facetious mixture of tedious reminiscence and fractious complaint. The occasional correspondent kept me honest as they say a—heroic task. Better than that. some of them kept me interested and directed my waning attention to new ideas that are better than the old and not just rediscovered versions academically resurrected.

One particularly fruitful month I had a letter from Moscow, where an ex-Family Medicine Programme panjandrum applied to the diplomatic community clinical skills honed in the Tasmanian hinterland and another from a colleague and neighbour now buried in the country two thousand miles or more from here.

The point of the second letter was that it is better to be buried in Wyndham, WA than cremated in metropolitan Melbourne, Vic. or Moscow, Russia for that matter.

He was a country gp (small letters), who viewed with some alarm a campaign to turn him into a Rural Doctor (capital letters). If I may quote him (that's another bonus from correspondents—suitably encouraged, they will write the column for you), he wrote in reference to a proposed rural medicine diploma:

> *The diploma is probably promulgated for all the right reasons but will perhaps generate a generation of diplomates too closely allied to a single way of thinking. But underlying it is an assumption—which I think should be challenged—that we are all the same and we all need highly organised and well-meaning chaps telling us what to do. Somehow the idea has been accepted that if you live more than two hours drive from some major town you are undereducated, underprivileged and desperately in need of help.*

I think there were two processes at work here that my correspondent rightly objected to.

First: the insidious and deadly process of irrelevant expertise mutating by academic replication into professional aggrandisement. It works like this.

Take any corner of a common subject, be it painting fence posts or treating umbilici, or as in the present case, looking after people on your own. Since it is a corner, it is necessarily darker than the middle of the room and sooner or later some honest fellow will be moved to light it up and announce to a largely indifferent world what dust and disaster they have found. Somewhere, someone else who has made the same discovery, but in silence, responds and a Society of Corner Watchers is formed with a monthly newsletter, an annual subscription and weekend seminars in tax-efficient hideaways, where the faithful chide their blinder colleagues, petition a neglectful government and alert the ever-watchful press. Add a disappointed academic, a disenchanted practitioner and a besieged politician and the thing is done—another college, another working party, another string of letters have arrived.

Worse still, the corner watchers exclude everybody else. The fence posts, however painted, now exclude the rest of us; the umbilici are on display only to the qualified gaze of the accredited.

'You might', 'you should', 'you ought', 'you must', are a familiar litany to anybody who has been in the game long enough but when it becomes 'you mustn't' then the fun begins. 'Says who?' 'The Professor' 'The Professor of what? 'Rural Medicine' 'Where is he/she? 'In Canberra.'

Second (I hadn't forgotten), what's different about medicine in the country? Professional isolation, poor medical facilities and restricted social amenities. But, as my correspondent pointed out, anyone with normal eyesight or serviceable reading glasses can keep themselves abreast of those professional topics they need to know about. Their postgraduate syllabus is written by their patients and their circumstances. They may enjoy the luxury of no competition, but they pay for it with necessary study, if only in self-defence.

Furthermore, anyone with a telephone should be able to call on city colleagues when they have need of them. A diploma course in how to advise the lone GP might have more relevance.

Facilities, whether in town or in the country, begin with men and women, not bricks and mortar, and with hands and heads and senses. What use is a scalpel in an uncertain or unsteady hand? If rural medicine will make available the essential technical skills for those whose isolation demands them, more power to it.

If metropolitan and academic medicine will allow their country cousins into those corners of their private pastures they may need to graze, embrace the revolutionary principle of limited scope for acceptable (even diplomatised) skills, so much the better.

And if we spoilt city slickers can help to ease the country doctor's burden, not by lectures in provincial centres but by practical help, even doing the occasional locum, better still.

But are we good enough? Are we so accustomed to the cushion of an after-hours service, the soft option of referral, the resigned surrender to so many others who seek to do our work or tell us how to do it? Do we still have the confidence and surety to handle emergencies other than by summoning an ambulance? Can we balance a clinical equation that adds 'how long', 'how far' and 'how bad' to the standard factors? Can we achieve the necessary concern that sharpens judgment without the anxiety that distorts it, bear the responsibility we cannot share, make the decision and live with it as we must live with all whom it may affect? What course of lectures can teach that?

Why, you may ponder, does anyone but a saint, a genius or a drunkard choose to doctor in the sticks?

I'll leave the last word to the man from Wyndham.

'Some of us who live in the bush want to be there because it is actually nicer to live in a small community where everybody knows you, where you're a friend as well as a doctor. What we really need is the opportunity to access good medical advice and treatment when necessary and the freedom to deliver the medicine the people need.'

Not much to ask—with or without a diploma.

quality street

He's my oldest friend, so when we meet we can argue without rancour and disagree without being disagreeable. We don't meet often and since we follow the same calling it follows that when we do, somewhere around the second glass of the evening, we drift into reminiscence or shop. We are agreed that we couldn't work together for more than 10 minutes, but we share, up to a point, a common outlook about the job we do. One recent evening we were discussing his whisky and the whole vexed question of quality assurance.

I'm for it, in principle anyway, although I will admit to qualms when attempting to defend my antique practices against the polite derision of younger, better-instructed colleagues. As the glasses fell, the voices rose and by bedtime we parted as so often before, wholly convinced of our unassailably correct but divergent views and woke our respective wives to repeat our arguments.

This argument lasted into the next day until, over the barbecue, my old friend said, 'All right, I'll take you to meet a friend of mine'. It was a man for whom he regularly deputised, whose practice he knew as only a long-time locum can and who saw quality assurance as a beguiling device to ensnare general practice in the nets of a malevolent bureaucracy and nothing else. Next day we went.

Picture a tiny town in rural NSW, population 500 or thereabouts, and a man in early middle age, a local son, long-time local doctor to that little place and a wide surrounding hinterland of mountains, cattle runs and lofty stands of timber. He was doctor of first and last and only contact to a scattered population of farmers, graziers and timbermen and a sizeable community of Aborigines. He was being torn, as so many country doctors are, between the claims of his patients and the needs of his family now outgrowing the local school. There was a price in family separation that he did not wish to pay and a cost in cash that an income, restricted by regulation designed for the control of city entrepreneurs, could not sustain.

He had successfully reversed a decision taken in a Sydney office half a thousand miles away to close the little hospital that was the most useful tool in his bulging doctor's bag. He had ruefully accepted the withdrawal of surgery, anaesthetics, obstetrics and radiology, also decreed by experts he had never seen and who, it may be inferred, knew and cared nothing of him and the realities of his working life.

He spoke of his Aboriginal patients with an unsentimental understanding. He accepted (as few of us do) their conception of 'soon' as 'maybe', 'tomorrow' as 'next time I'm in town' and 'now' as 'when dad gets back from the pub with the car'. He talked of the rise of venereal disease among these people, the re-emergence of syphilis as a diagnostic possibility and the high proportion of cerebrovascular involvement that he had come across. Should he lumbar puncture every new case, or treat every one on the assumption that they might have it? The professors to whom he wrote didn't know and the watch-dogs of the public purse would only see it as overservicing. His own studies had been hijacked by the health department. He no longer had a place in the survey of a problem he had been the first to recognise.

He described himself as a human biologist, a rarity he thought in medical practice, although I have always thought the old word 'naturalist' exactly describes the essence of general practice. Patient observation, careful recording, accurate description and a genuine sympathy for those we study, is surely what we ought to be about.

I knew that he had spent time in Antarctica, had even enriched the scientific literature on Emperor Penguins. I learnt that afternoon that on his return from the South Pole he had gone back to being a resident to acquaint himself with recent developments and equip himself for rural isolation.

And now he was pondering migration to a city where good schools were close at hand and syphilitics were tidied quietly away into special clinics. I wondered what city could give this man the role he now adorned, the stimulus he sought or the recognition he deserved. Even more I wondered how you would classify or estimate the worth of so singular a colleague. Because, and I am proud to think it, he is just that—a colleague. Just another GP, a provider number[4], a health care professional to be educated by readers in community medicine, admonished by committees 'who only want to help him', wooed with practice grants and excluded from any territory that another discipline has staked out for itself.

For all that, I could not give my friend the victory that evening or admit defeat even on the testimony of such a witness. There is a place for quality assurance. We do not all bring such single-minded interest to our daily work. As Groucho Marx once put it, 'I don't want to belong to a club that lets in people like me'.

Lesser mortals need some more objective standard than the admiration of favoured patients and the approbation of the bank manager. But they are entitled to have some part in framing them. I am prepared to submit myself to the scrutiny of strangers, as long as they are fellow workers in the field, not imports from the lecture hall. We must set some practical measure of performance, if only for self-esteem and look critically at one another, if only for self defence—or watch each other's backs, at any rate.

There are and always will be, please God, men and women who cannot be compressed into the common mould, who create unsightly bulges in that seamless robe (so like a shroud), woven by the bureaucrats and classroom clinicians.

Eccentric? Yes, in the literal sense off-centre to the rest of us, not the centre, but paradoxically the core.

Out-of-step? Undoubtedly, but they march to a different music, less brazen maybe, but more certain of the destination.

One off? Unquestionably, but that has always been the glory of our trade. One appendix is much the same as another. It's the same spirochaete in Double Bay as in Arnhem Land, but the adolescent who remains after his appendix has been thrown away, the incautious philanderer purged of his social contagion—that's a different matter. In all the diversity of humankind, there is a place for a diversity of doctors.

But how can you and I, and we're the only ones that can or should, weigh the man I met in some objective balance? Only I suspect by watching him at work. Seeing the challenges he meets and the solutions he proposes to problems we will never meet. We may begin to wonder, as he does himself, how much longer he and his family will endure the pressure that every day, every term time, every bank statement brings. And ask ourselves: Who will take his place?

I won't tell you his name or where he lives, but I can tell you where to find him.

On quality street.

on second thoughts

'I wondered about a second opinion.'

It was a gentle, almost diffident, request from a lady whose first born I had delivered more years ago than either of us cared to remember. But I do remember the repeated monosyllabic expletive with which she mitigated the pangs of childbirth. Since that time, she has consulted me mostly on gynaecological occasions, but has relied for most of her care on my colleague in the neighbouring village where she lives.

Over the years we moved from childbirth to contraception to hormone replacement, her children (mine too, in a sense) from infancy to independence and she from housewife and mother to full-time teacher where her adult life had started.

It was this that brought her over to me. Her particular expertise was in the care of the rebellious, the neglected, the misfits and the rejects, whom society has taught only how to resist teaching.

One of her charges, it seemed, had expressed his point of view by throwing a bench at her. Happily, no obvious harm was done (no doubt that kind of job makes you quick on your feet) other than a minor loss of skin too big for a bandaid and too small for a graft, and she limped back to work undaunted the following morning. I wondered if her childbirth vocabulary had sprung to mind.

I don't know how the breach of discipline was healed, but the breach of epithelium alas was not, at least in the two months before she showed it to me. It's an awkward place the shin, especially the female shin, but I adopted my standard procedure—and then another—and then another. I sent her to a dermatologist, an erudite and witty man, but even he, deprived of his standard remedies already used in vain and unable to incriminate 'Avon' as he usually did, could only suggest a vascular surgeon.

Small beer indeed for a resecter of aneurisms and salvager of blackened limbs, but since he was too ethical to suggest another dermatologist and too fair-minded to advise a psychiatrist, he sent her back to me.

Hence the gentle request. My response, after that faint dismay and fainter guilt that all such requests provoke, was to ask, 'Whom did you have in mind?'

She named my colleague, my rival, that other doctor in another town with whom I shared her confidence. It took a millisecond or two to come to terms with this suggestion. After all, this man was one of my own kind, worse still, he was younger. Who was she to suggest that he might succeed where I had failed? Worst of all, what if he did? Then, resisting the urge to agree in that doubtful superior tone we use which means 'You're not only barmy, but ungrateful into the bargain, but I'm far too well-bred to say so', I yielded gracefully.

What's more, I did it properly. I thanked her, genuinely enough, for asking me first and there and then wrote him a letter, a proper letter of referral such as I send to any other consultant colleague. For that, in fact, was what he was. I outlined the problem, sketched in the background and sought his help.

Six or so weeks passed and he rang me up. He had cured the thing. He was modestly jubilant and faintly incredulous at an outcome neither of us—all three if you include the patient—had expected. He accepted my congratulations and concluded the conversation by saying 'So there's no need for her to come back to me any more and I've told her to come back to you'.

Why, as I used to remark in my courting days, don't we do this more often? Here we all are, so many from such diverse backgrounds, differing experiences, varied interests and expertise. Why don't we share it around, give credit where it is due, confess our particular deficiencies and supply those of others where we can? Is it jealousy, suspicion, simple greed or complex pride that strangles an honest call for help or a disinterested offer?

An ignoble search for quality assurance points takes me once a fortnight to a small group of colleagues who meet to exchange knowledge rather than absorb it from outside. At the most there's only 10 of us, but varied skills are encompassed. I have learnt about diving medicine, tricky knees and shoulders, headaches and acupuncture, hirsutism and senile dementia. All from colleagues, all with something fresh to say and all of whom have at least temporarily increased my dwindling stock of knowledge. If I have learnt nothing else, I now know who to ask and where to find out.

More important still, I know where to send my problems, secure in the knowledge that the recipient understands the background from which they spring, the unique features of family medicine and the practical solutions applicable to that setting. I also dare to believe that my patients will come back to me.

None of us claims omniscience or aspire to that heroic absurdity 'total patient care', a phrase that usually translates to care by a committee all of whose members push their barrows in diverging directions. At best we attempt care of the total patient, which is rather like conducting an orchestra of soloists whose pitch and rhythm rarely harmonise.

Among ourselves there is a certain cynicism about our specialist brethren, to balance no doubt a reciprocal scorn of us, but it is nothing to the contempt we nourish for fellow family doctors with differing and perhaps greater skills. The phrase 'Why they're only a GP' is not restricted to the laity. But there is a vast library of knowledge, skill and wisdom to which the only subscription is an open mind.

Am I proposing yet another tier of self-appointed pseudo-specialists, another confederation of empire builders, another fragment in a system already, God knows, fragmented enough? Not really. There is a set of problems peculiar to general practice that GPs are best fitted to solve. All it takes is trust, mutual respect, professional integrity and a certain humility.

We could use that in other places too.

a plague on all our houses

After the euphoria of qualifying has passed and you shrink slowly back to standard human dimensions, after you have joined the Medical Defence Union and practised adding the magic letters to your signature on secret scraps of paper, you come, rather heavily, down to earth.

I was not one of the favoured few invited to stay on at the alma mater en route for specialist stardom. So, with the mediocre majority I looked for work and after flirting with far away places and improbable appointments found myself reporting to an erstwhile fever hospital on the lower reaches of the Thames, which had by a stroke of the administrative pen become an acute general hospital.

It was an extraordinary place, a series of pavilions linked by covered pathways, hidden behind a forbidding perimeter of high stone walls. The only access was through iron gates guarded by a porter who booked you in and out, presumably to ensure that no one stole away with one of the plagues happily incubating within. There were one or two lepers and the occasional malaria patient fresh from Africa secreted in odd, unvisited corners; a building full of children with tuberculous meningitis; and sundry other blocks given over to the usual hospital services.

The consultant staff included three elderly experts who for 30 years had painted chicken pox with gentian violet and tonsillitis with Mandels paint and seemed unaware of the disappearance of diphtheria. At the flash of a yellow flag they would put to sea to board some passing P&O liner in search of doubtful vesicles, while cursing nurses made up the beds in the smallpox section and sweating residents thumbed ancient texts on the management of dread diseases which now, thank God, have largely disappeared.

The whole place was, like the lunatic asylums of the last century and the sanatoria of this century, a monument to dead medicine, a crumbling rampart against a siege long since lifted.

I grew up in the era when infectious disease was of no consequence in civilised places. We had antibiotics to make the world safe for hypertension, coronary disease, peptic ulcers and lung cancer.

There were occasional panics. Polio closed the swimming pools and filled the iron lungs for a while and exotics intruded now and again from Africa. The Marburg virus and Lassa fever joined Rocky Mountain spotted fever and scrub typhus on the honours list of differential diagnosis. The American legion popped up unexpectedly from time to time, but had the grace to respond (mostly) to erythromycin.

Then, all of a sudden, there came an infection we couldn't cure. What started as a footnote in the journals invaded the bathhouses of San Francisco and the blood banks of the world. Scientific challenge or divine retribution, the AIDS virus has infected thousands of bodies and millions of minds. It has stirred governments and scared people all over. And we, the carers, are not immune.

I wonder what our medieval colleagues must have thought as the Black Death swept across Europe, wiping out cities and re-writing history. Did they too succumb to xenophobia, that pathological dread of strangers black, white or yellow, loathsome and different from themselves? Will we put figurative crosses on the doors of the afflicted? Will some municipal union push out the charnel carts crying 'Bring out your dead'?

I believe not. There is still in every caring trade a basic sense of responsibility to others. (I typed 'outers' at first—a better word, perhaps.) We still accept the hazards no less than the dignities of our commitment. But we also have a right to such rational protection as is possible. I do not see routine screening as an invasion of privacy but simply as sensible prevention. I am sworn to treat you. Is it too much to ask that you will do your part to protect me? I will not pass on my knowledge to outsiders. I am used to keeping secrets.

The volunteers who of their generosity give blood for others accept their obligation not to harm. If the objection to screening is that it demeans the screened and perhaps advertises their condition, then the alternative is to assume that all who pass under our hands are infected; to isolate, restrict surgery to survival care and carry the no-touch technique to the theatre, ward—and the consulting room.

The plague will pass, as other plagues have passed, and like them it will leave scars behind. No doubt our descendants will smile at our ignorance and chide our folly.

But, I hope that in the meantime we will behave with the courage and dignity of our forebears and that my last job won't be back in that fever hospital.

——————————— valedictory

valedictory

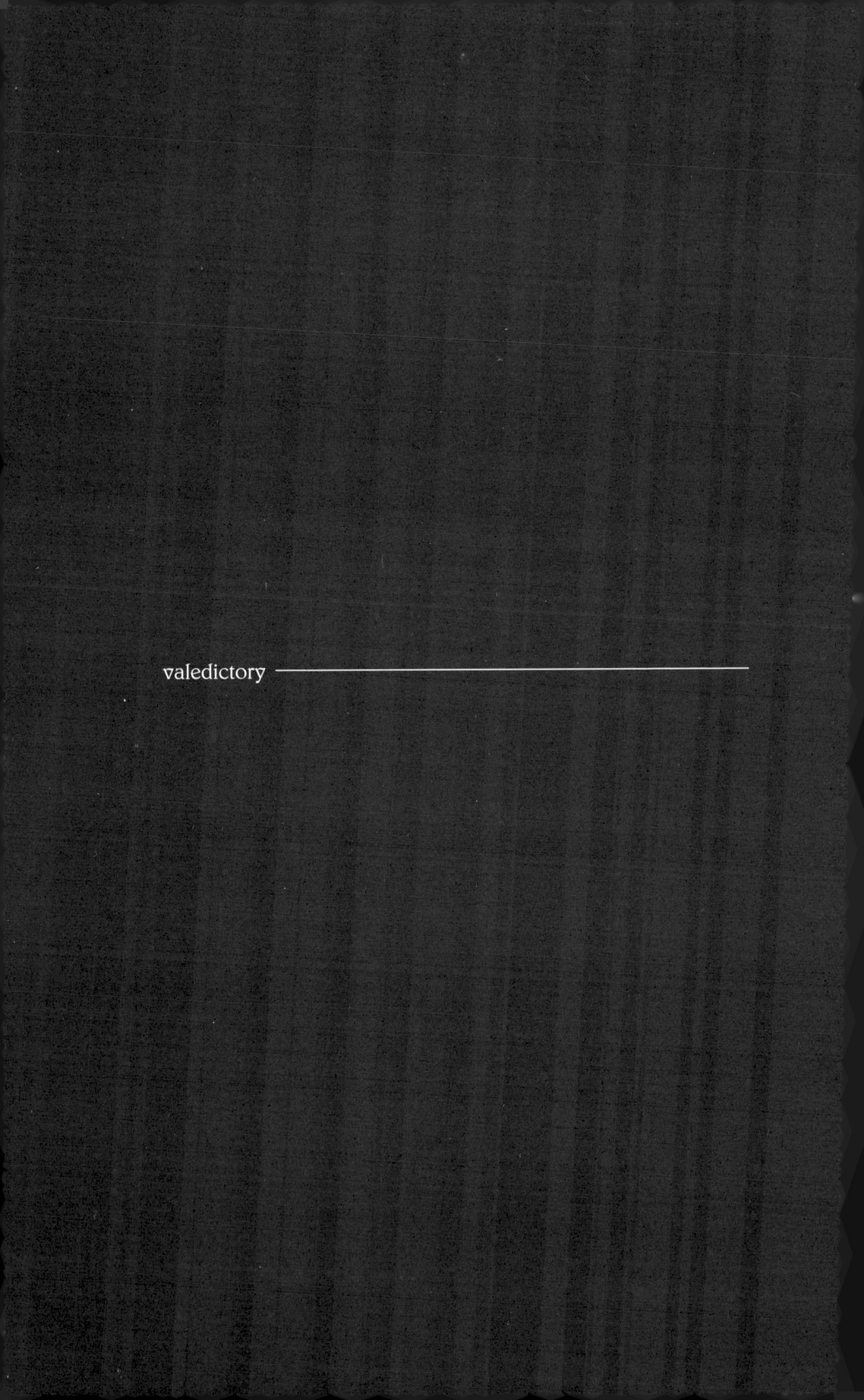

valedictory

The buses of my youth had an open platform at the back, vertically divided by a pole which served, in theory, to separate those entering from those alighting. It also functioned as a goal for those foolish or athletic enough to attempt the forbidden practice of entering a moving vehicle.

So often I remember the conductor watching a laggard sprinting for his stationary conveyance, only to give the signal for departure four or five paces before he reached it. I should here explain that in that era of the 'new look' and hobble skirts, it was an exclusively male pursuit. A woman could hardly board, let alone chase, a London bus.

What followed was something between melodrama, sport and ritual immolation. The young athlete, among whom I counted myself in those distant days, lengthened his stride, accelerated his pace, lunged for the departing pole and if successful, had won the first set. He was by now so doubled up that his legs could not cover the lengthening gap without serious risk of abrasion to the shin, humiliation to the soul, an abrupt descent into the gutter and naturally a loss of game, set and match.

The determined, however, hung on, quickened their pace and tried to match one human against 97 horse power in a race that only death, dyspnoea or traffic lights could terminate. An interested gallery of passengers offered advice and encouragement, while a critical conductor adjudicated with professional detachment. If, as usually happened, the breathless aspirant gave up the struggle, it was not unknown for a fair-minded conductor to stop the bus and help him aboard.

It seems to me that my professional life can in some respects be likened to that harmless pastime. I too have nearly missed so many buses, have sprinted with increasing effort to leap aboard some vehicle in which most of my colleagues are already smugly seated. Alas, no one ever rang the bell to let me on, but once in a while the bus was discovered to be going in the wrong direction and I saved myself an unnecessary journey. At least I was able to remind myself that 'there's always another bus'.

Now 40 years on, I am beginning to believe that perhaps for me there isn't.

What do I remember, waiting at the deserted stop, of the succession of clinical journeys I have taken? So many destinations reached by accident or never reached at all, so many different buses shabby or sleek, noisy or silent, standing room only or with a solitary passenger. Even the notices have changed. In the era of tubercle you were forbidden to spit; in the age of lung cancer you are banned from smoking.

Yet so many of these journeys seem, in retrospect, to have been circular. I boarded in the early antibiotic age when we told ourselves that bacterial disease would shortly disappear in a barrage of magic bullets. Now I read of wily staphs that keep one jump ahead, erstwhile friendly streps that are armed, dangerous and bullet proof.

I grew up to dread the summer months when polio closed the swimming pools and filled the iron lungs, those clanking tanks on which a life depended. I saw it disappear as vaccines expunged it from the diagnostic list. I marvelled at the disappearance of smallpox, little knowing what was yet to come from Africa. I applauded the control of malaria, fleeting and uncertain as it has proved to be. I watched almost with regret the taming of measles, that biennial certainty of every general practice.

Where now are the wards of rheumatic heart disease—mitrals on this floor, aortics upstairs, the refill clinics for artificial pneumothoraces, the ECT sessions, the twice weekly carnage of Ts and As? Gone maybe, but replaced. For every question answered, a newer more complex one is posed. As the understanding of immunology has blossomed, its greatest challenge multiplies until it shadows half the world. For every tonsil saved, another grommet is inserted. No sooner do we crack the genetic code than a new pollutant menaces it in our polluted world.

The asylums are empty but the dependency units have a two-month waiting list and the Salvation Army is almost overwhelmed. I have abandoned the inaccuracy of chronic bronchitis for the imprecision of COAD and seen the varieties of hepatitis double with more to come (and against all of which, apparently, it is essential to vaccinate school teachers). I have watched the surgeons annex coronary artery disease and the physicians take out a lien on peptic ulcers. I have struggled through a maze of acronyms and initials until I didn't know whether it was the disease or the author who was thus described.

I have changed sides at least three times, usually too late, in the wavering battle between bronchodilator and steroid and confirmed my opinion that asthma is always worse here than it is there, always more common now than it was then. I have learnt that status anginosus is a myth—and crescendo angina a grim reality. I have seen digoxin pass from good to bad, to sometimes quite useful. It was once negligent not to screen your antenatal patients for syphilis; now it's almost actionable to screen them for AIDS.

I started with a typewriter; I shall finish, thank God, with a word processor. I began as a humble helper clinging to the skirts of experts, a lowly GP too shy to ask questions, too overawed to disagree. Now I see my colleagues, confident and determined, being offered control of the purse strings. I set out alone and leave an impressive company beginning to find its voice and savour its power.

Some things haven't changed. The tolerance, patience and unfailing courtesy of a succession of medical editors and their administrative staff who have sheltered this scrawny strident chicken beneath their eagle wings; the odd message from the great Out There of readers—the occasional bouquet from Queensland, a well-directed broadside from New South Wales, a raspberry from Adelaide and a distant cheer from the Northern Territory; the trauma of a blank sheet of paper and the doubtful pleasure of filling it. I have made so many friends I have never seen, so many critics (but never an enemy—what writer calls his readers that) I would never otherwise have known. The anxious mums I once reassured are grandmothers now, but still in need of reassurance. For all the anodynes and expert counsel nothing wholly eases the pain of dying or the telling of bad news. I may have learnt to replace the anxious solicitude of the young doctor with the practised detachment of the old, but to what benefit?

Now younger colleagues and ever younger, it seems, consultants listen with polite inattention to my tedious clinical reminiscences and deal kindly with my antique misconceptions. When I look up from the desk I sometimes catch that half-quizzical, half-affectionate glance from a patient that reads 'Bless him—the poor old sod'. Former patients slip pass me in the corridor en route to my fresher, better instructed partners. Balint talked long ago of the drug 'doctor'. This one I fear has just about reached his 'use by date'. Now would be the time to quit, if not the job, at least writing about it.

So my peers and partners, loyal staff and helpful betters, patient publishers and unseen readers, my loyal/fickle, generous/grudging, grateful/ungrateful, thoughtful/inconsiderate patients who have taught me my trade and let me briefly into their lives mostly, I hope, for their benefit as well as mine, it's time to ring the bell and let me off.

Thank you all for your company, your good counsel and even better friendship.

Should you ever be inclined to look me up you'll find me where I now belong. Among the back numbers.

notes and references

1 Parker, O.B. 'On our selection: predictors of medical school success', *Medical Journal of Australia,* No. 156, 7 June 1993, p. 747 et seq.
2 For those who still read references you'll find it in *The Sign of the Four* by that failed GP and still successful author, Arthur Conan Doyle.
3 'The Thing', republished in the Everyman Library Stories, *Essays and Poems,* by G. K. Chesterton, J. M. Dent & Sons, London, 1935.
4 Provider number: the number which identifies each doctor entitled to provide professional services under the Australian Commonwealth Government's health care system.